COPYCAT RECIPES MAKING

A Complete Cookbook for making American and Mexican restaurants' favorite dishes at home saving your money. Over 140 recipes for breakfasts, appetizers, soups, burgers, juices, and desserts to improve your life.

MELANIE STEVIE

TABLE OF CONTENTS

INTRODUCTION

Congratulations on purchasing *Copycat Recipes Making,* and thank you for doing so.

You will not be able to find someone who does not like to go out and enjoy some great food at fine-dine cafes and restaurants every once in a while. It might be a family dinner night or a special outing with a close friend. Not only that, but we also love to get some breakfast on our way to our office from some cafes and restaurants whenever we do not get enough time to prepare our breakfast. Many a time, we do not feel like cooking or going to a restaurant. So, we order our favorite dishes at our home to fulfill our cravings. However, many people think that the dishes from our favorite restaurants cannot be made or prepared in our home kitchen. That is what makes people visit their favorite restaurants to enjoy their favorite meals. But, no matter which restaurant you prefer, be it Applebee's or Olive Garden, you can easily prepare your favorite dishes simply by taking the help of copycat recipes.

With copycat recipes by your side, you will no longer need to wait in long queues for enjoying some tasty pizza or spend a lot of money on food as you can prepare them at your home kitchen at about half the price. The ingredients that are used for preparing the copycat recipes are very simple, along with super easy steps. Dining out every now and then is a favorite pass time for many people. But, that will not only be affecting your wallet but your waistline as well. According to some reports published by the United States Healthful Food Council, an average adult from the USA buys a meal or a snack from a restaurant or a café for almost six times each week. Also, about thirty percent of children have been found to consume various types of fast foods during any day of the week.

Depending on outside food has different types of consequences. The intake of dietary fibers gets reduced by half with an increase in the total percentage of trans fat, saturated fat, sodium, and various other additives. Most of these come from fast foods and sweetened beverages such as soda. However, when you shift your focus from restaurants and fast food joints and concentrate on home-cooked foods, you can easily maintain your health and keep a check on your expenditures. But, that does not mean you cannot enjoy the taste of restaurant foods. Luckily, with the help of copycat recipes, you can maintain a healthy lifestyle without compromising your favorite tastes.

With the help of copycat recipes, you can maintain the cooking methods and great control over the ingredients that you are going to use. All these are essential for establishing a healthy lifestyle. Let's have a look at some of the benefits of homemade food.

- **Great control over the portions:** When you decide to cook your favorite food at home, it will become easier for you to maintain the food amount that you are going to eat. The fast-food joints and restaurants tend to offer you huge portions of food to provide the appearance of great value. It can easily urge you to overeat. But, when you cook at home, there is no pressure to finish all that you have on the plate. In case the amount of food is more than you can actually eat, you can always store it in the refrigerator for later consumption. This way, you can have the proper amount of food along with less wastage of money.

- **Proper control over food hygiene and safety:** It has been found that there more than 260 types of foodborne diseases. Every year, almost one in every five people tends to fall prey to them. When you cook your favorite dishes at home, you can easily maintain safety and food hygiene to prepare a healthy meal.

- **A great option for maintaining nutrition:** When you decide to cook at home, there are various ways to maintain the nutrition content of the meals. For example, you can opt for steaming or grilling your food items in place of frying them for effectively cutting down the content of fat. You will be able to preserve the maximum percentage of the nutritional value of the prepared food items.

- **A great family time:** Cooking at home can help you to maintain a great family time. You can divide the work between various family members and get indulged in cooking together. Also, dining with the family members at home has been linked to less percentage of substance abuse within any kind of family.

In this book, you will find various copycat recipes from your favorite restaurants in the USA and various cities in Mexico. Whether you want some tasty burgers from McDonald's or enjoy some Italian specialties from Olive Garden, you will find everything you need in this book.

There are plenty of books on this subject on the market, thanks again for choosing this one! Every effort was made to ensure it is full of as much useful information as possible; please enjoy!

PART 1:
COPYCAT RECIPES
FROM USA

The USA is often regarded as the hub of some of the most renowned restaurants and eating hubs where you can enjoy every meal of the day. In this section, you will find various recipes from some of the USA's top restaurants that can be made easily at your home kitchen.

CHAPTER 1:
BREAKFAST RECIPES

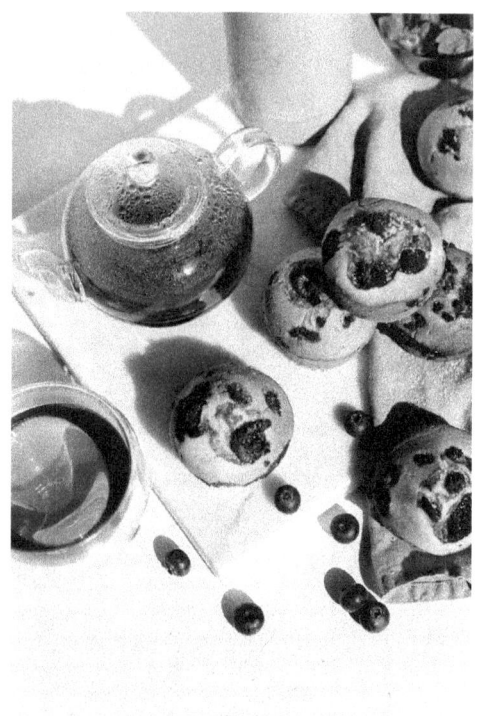

Feta and Spinach Wrap (Starbucks)

Total Prep & Cooking Time: Fifteen minutes

Yields: Two servings

Nutrition Facts: Calories: 192.3 | Protein: 13.6g | Carbs: 17.8g | Fat: 8.9g | Fiber: 10.9g

Ingredients

- Two large tortillas

- Two egg whites

- Half cup of spinach

- Eight sun-dried tomatoes (chopped)

- Four tbsps. of feta (crumbled)

- One tsp. of salt

- One and a half tsp. of black pepper (ground)

Method:

1. Take a non-stick pan. Heat some oil in it. Add the egg whites and cook for two minutes on each side. Fold the egg whites and remove from heat.

2. Add the spinach to the pan. Cook for two minutes until wilted.

3. Take a parchment paper and place the tortillas; add the cooked egg whites, sun-dried tomatoes, spinach, along with the crumbled feta. Add pepper and salt according to taste.

4. Wrap the tortillas and seal the ends.

5. Place the wraps in a pan and grill them for five minutes.

6. Before serving, cut the wraps in half.

Egg, Bacon, And Gouda Sandwich (Starbucks)

Total Prep & Cooking Time: Thirty minutes

Yields: Two servings

Nutrition Facts: Calories: 380.2 | Protein: 21.3g | Carbs: 40.5g | Fat: 12.3g | Fiber: 1.2g

Ingredients

- Two ciabatta rolls (small, sliced)

- Two slices of Gouda cheese

- Two large eggs

- Two slices of bacon (cooked)

Method:

1. Take an iron skillet and add one tsp. of oil in it. Add the eggs. Scramble them on low flame for two minutes.

2. Arrange the bottom parts of the ciabatta rolls on a baking tray.

3. Add cooked eggs, bacon, along with Gouda. Add the other half of the rolls.

4. Cook for twenty seconds until the cheese melts.

5. Serve hot.

Blueberry Muffins (Starbucks)

Total Prep & Cooking Time: Fifty minutes

Yields: Twenty-four servings

Nutrition Facts: Calories: 190.3 | Protein: 2.1g | Carbs: 24.6g | Fat: 6.3g | Fiber: 1.3g

Ingredients

For the topping:

- One cup of flour
- Half cup of granulated sugar
- One-fourth tsp. of salt
- Five tbsps. of butter (unsalted, melted)

For the muffins:

- Two large eggs
- One cup of granulated sugar
- Half cup of oil
- One tsp. of each
  - Baking soda
  - White vinegar
- One tbsp. of vanilla extract

- Half tsp. of salt

- One and a half cup of sour cream

- Two cups of flour

- One-third cup of blueberries

Method:

1. Heat your oven at one-hundred and seventy-five degrees Celsius. Line a muffin pan with baking cups.

2. Add all the listed topping ingredients in a bowl. Mix well and keep aside.

3. Crack the eggs in a large bowl. Beat the eggs using a hand blender. Mix for two minutes until frothy and thick; add oil and sugar. Mix for two minutes.

4. Add vinegar, vanilla extract, salt, and baking soda; add the sour cream along with the flour. Use a spatula for stirring the mixture. Add the blueberries and mix again.

5. Fill the baking cups with the muffin mixture. Top the muffin cups with the prepared topping. Bake for twenty minutes.

6. Let the muffins rest in the oven for five minutes.

7. Serve warm or at room temperature.

Egg And Sausage McMuffin (McDonald's)

Total Prep & Cooking Time: Thirty minutes

Yields: Four servings

Nutrition Facts: Calories: 451.3 | Protein: 12.3g | Carbs: 60.3g | Fat: 14.3g | Fiber: 2.9g

Ingredients

For the sausage patties:

- Five-hundred grams of pork (ground)

- Half tsp. of dried sage (ground)

- One-third tsp. of thyme (dried)

- One tsp. of onion powder

- Three-fourth tsp. of each

    - Salt

    - Black pepper

- Two tsps. of sugar

For the muffins:

- Two tbsps. of oil

- Four large eggs

- Four English muffins

- Four cheese slices

Method:

1. Preheat your oven at one-hundred and thirty degrees Celsius.

2. Add the muffins on a baking sheet by cutting them in halves. Top the muffin slices with cheese and bake.

3. Mix the ingredients for the patties in a large bowl. Combine well.

4. Use your hands to shape four equal-sized patties.

5. Heat some oil in a skillet. Add the patties. Cook the patties for three minutes on both sides.

6. Heat a pan; add some oil in it. Place egg rings on the pan. Crack the eggs in the rings and cook them for two minutes.

7. Arrange the muffins on a working surface. Add sausage patties and top with eggs. Top with the other halves of the muffins.

8. Serve hot.

Hash Browns (McDonald's)

Total Prep & Cooking Time: Thirty minutes

Yields: Six servings

Nutrition Facts: Calories: 380 | Protein: 4.9g | Carbs: 29.3g | Fat: 27.5g | Fiber: 3.2g

Ingredients

- Four large potatoes (parboiled, peeled, grated)
- One large egg
- One-third cup of flour
- Salt (for seasoning)
- One tsp. of black pepper (ground)
- Two tbsps. of butter (softened)
- Oil (for frying)

Method:

1. Combine grated potatoes, flour, egg, pepper, butter, and salt in a bowl. Mix well. Use your hands to make six equal-sized hash browns.

2. Add oil in a pan. Add the hash browns and cook for three minutes on each side.

3. Serve hot.

Sugar Glazed Donuts (Krispy Kreme)

Total Prep & Cooking Time: One hour and thirty minutes

Yields: Four servings

Nutrition Facts: Calories: 451.3 | Protein: 12.3g | Carbs: 60.3g | Fat: 14.3g | Fiber: 2.9g

Ingredients

For the glaze:

- Four cups of powdered sugar
- Half cup of milk
- One pinch of salt

For the donuts:

- Two cups of whole milk
- Three tsps. of instant yeast
- Two large eggs
- Eight tbsps. of butter (unsalted)
- One-fourth cup of granulated sugar
- One tsp. of salt
- Five cups of bread flour

- Oil (to fry)

Method:

1. Microwave the milk for forty seconds. Add the yeast and stir well. Let the milk mixture sit for five minutes until foam forms on top.

2. Add eggs, sugar, salt, and butter. Use a mixer for combining the ingredients. Add flour and mix again. Let the dough sit for thirty minutes.

3. Pour the dough in a floured working surface. Knead again. Roll the dough into a thickness of half-inch. Use a donut cutter for cutting the donuts.

4. Arrange the donut rounds in a baking tray and cover them with a kitchen towel. Let them sit for twenty minutes.

5. Heat oil in a pan. Add the donuts and fry for forty seconds on each side.

6. Mix together the listed glaze ingredients in a bowl.

7. Start dipping one side of the donuts into the prepared glaze. Use a fork for flipping them over.

8. Place the donuts on a cooling rack. Let them sit for fifteen minutes.

Banana Pancakes (Denny's)

Total Prep & Cooking Time: Forty minutes

Yields: Eight servings

Nutrition Facts: Calories: 180.2 | Protein: 6.5g | Carbs: 30.1g | Fat: 4.2g | Fiber: 2.9g

Ingredients

- One cup of each
    - Flour
    - Wheat flour
- Four tsps. of baking powder
- One tsp. of cinnamon (ground)
- Half tsp. of salt
- Two large eggs
- Two cups of milk (fat-free)
- Two-third cup of a ripe banana (mashed)
- One tbsp. of each
    - Maple syrup
    - Olive oil
- One-third tsp. of vanilla extract

Method:

1. Mix the first five ingredients in a large bowl.

2. In another bowl, mix milk, eggs, oil, banana, vanilla extract, and syrup. Combine well and add this mixture to the mixture of flour.

3. Heat a pan. Use a cooking spray for greasing the pan. Add one-fourth cup of batter in the pan. Cook for five minutes on each side.

4. Top with sliced bananas and serve.

Swiss Cheese And Ham Omelet (Denny's)

Total Prep & Cooking Time: Twenty minutes

Yields: Two servings

Nutrition Facts: Calories: 501.3 | Protein: 31.6g | Carbs: 4.6g | Fat: 36.9g | Fiber: 0.6g

Ingredients

- One tbsp. of butter

- Four large eggs

- Six tbsps. of water

- One tsp. of salt

- Two tsps. of black pepper (ground)

- One cup of cooked ham (cubed)

- One and a half cup of Swiss cheese (shredded)

Method:

1. Whisk together eggs, salt, pepper, and water in a bowl.

2. Heat an iron skillet; add some oil. Pour the egg mixture in the skillet.

3. Cook the eggs for two minutes. Add ham cubes and sprinkle shredded cheese from the top.

4. Fold the omelet and flip. Cook for two minutes.

5. Cut the omelet in half. Serve hot.

Egg In A Basket (Cracker Barrel)

Total Prep & Cooking Time: Twenty minutes

Yields: Two servings

Nutrition Facts: Calories: 341.3 | Protein: 11.3g | Carbs: 32.5g | Fat: 17.4g | Fiber: 1.6g

Ingredients

- Two slices of sourdough bread

- Two tbsps. of butter

- Two large eggs

- Pepper and salt (for seasoning)

Method:

1. Take a cookie cutter for cutting out a circle from the center of the bread slices.

2. Spread the butter on each side of the bread.

3. Heat a skillet and add the bread slices.

4. Crack the eggs in the cutout circle. Add pepper and salt. Cook for two minutes.

5. Flip the bread slices and cook for one minute.

6. Serve hot.

Cheesy Egg And Veggie bake (IHOP)

Total Prep & Cooking Time: One hour

Yields: Ten servings

Nutrition Facts: Calories: 216.3 | Protein: 16.3g | Carbs: 4.6g | Fat: 15.2g | Fiber: 1.2g

Ingredients

- Two tbsps. of olive oil
- Four ounces of mushrooms (cremini)
- One cup of broccoli florets
- Half red bell pepper (chopped)
- One-fourth red onion (chopped)
- Twelve spears of asparagus
- Twelve large eggs
- Half cup of milk (whole)
- One tsp. of salt
- One-fourth tsp. of black pepper (ground)
- Four ounces of each
  - Cheddar cheese (shredded)
  - Mozzarella cheese (shredded)

- Two ounces of parmesan cheese (grated)

Method:

1. Preheat your oven at one-hundred and seventy degrees Celsius.

2. Take a casserole dish and grease it using cooking spray.

3. Slice the cremini mushrooms. Chop the florets of broccoli and asparagus.

4. Add olive oil in a large iron skillet. Add all the veggies and cook for eight minutes.

5. Whisk together milk, eggs, black, pepper, and salt in a large bowl. Add the cooked veggies along with the shredded cheese. Mix well.

6. Pour the mixture into the greased casserole.

7. Bake for forty minutes.

8. Use a sharp knife for cutting the casserole in squares and serve hot.

CHAPTER 2: SNACK AND SIDE DISH RECIPES

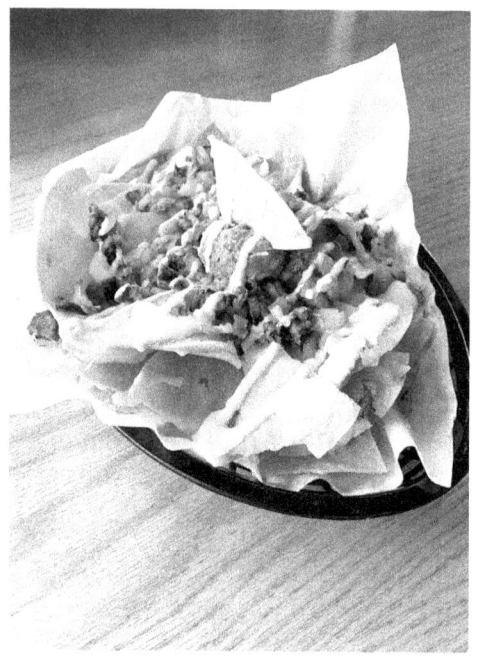

Cheddar And Bacon Potato Skins (TGI Friday's)

Total Prep & Cooking Time: Thirty minutes

Yields: Eight servings

Nutrition Facts: Calories: 310.3 | Protein: 12.2g | Carbs: 30.4g | Fat: 17.2g | Fiber: 4.1g

Ingredients

- Four large potatoes (baked)

- Three tbsps. of canola oil

- One tbsp. of parmesan cheese

- Half tsp. of salt

- One-fourth tsp. of each

  o Paprika

  o Garlic powder

- One-eighth tsp. of pepper

- Eight strips of bacon (cooked, crumbled)

- Two cups of cheddar cheese (shredded)

- Half cup of sour cream

- Four green onions (sliced)

Method:

1. Preheat your oven at two-hundred degrees Celsius.

2. Cut the baked potatoes in half; use a spoon for scooping out the pulp. Leave behind about one-fourth inch of the pulp.

3. Arrange the potato skins of a baking tray.

4. Mix oil, parmesan cheese, salt, garlic powder, paprika, pepper, and crumbled bacon.

5. Brush the oil mixture over the potato skins.

6. Bake for seven minutes.

7. Add cheddar cheese and leftover bacon inside the potato skin. Bake for two minutes.

8. Add onions and sour cream. Serve immediately.

Spinach Florentine Flatbread (TGI Friday's)

Total Prep & Cooking Time: Fifty minutes

Yields: Six servings

Nutrition Facts: Calories: 285.9 | Protein: 14.2g | Carbs: 30.3g | Fat: 11.3g | Fiber: 5.2g

Ingredients

- One cup of flour (whole wheat)

- One tsp. of baking powder

- One-fourth tsp. of salt

- Half tsp. of each

    o Basil (dried)

    o Parsley flakes

    o Oregano

- Three-fourth cup of beer

For the toppings:

- One tsp. of olive oil

- One clove of garlic (minced)

- Two cups of each

    o Baby spinach

- o   Italian cheese blend

- One can of artichoke hearts (drained, chopped)

- Two tomatoes (chopped)

- Two tbsps. of basil (sliced)

Method:

1. Preheat your oven at two-hundred degrees Celsius.

2. In a small bowl, combine flour, baking powder, salt, and dried herbs. Add the beer and stir well.

3. Place the dough on a flat surface with some flour. Knead properly. Press the dough for fitting a pizza pan of twelve inches. Bake for eight minutes.

4. Combine garlic and oil. Add the mixture over the crust.

5. Add half a cup of cheese all over the crust. Arrange artichoke, spinach, and tomatoes. Top with the remaining cheese.

6. Bake for ten minutes.

7. Slice with the help of a knife and sprinkle basil from the top.

8. Serve hot.

Loaded Chicken Nachos (TGI Friday's)

Total Prep & Cooking Time: Forty-five minutes

Yields: Sixteen servings

Nutrition Facts: Calories: 212.6 | Protein: 11.2g | Carbs: 13.4g | Fat: 12.3g | Fiber: 2.2g

Ingredients

- Two sweet red peppers (diced)

- One green pepper (diced)

- Three tsps. of canola oil

- One can of black beans (rinsed)

- One tsp. of each

  o Oregano (dried)

  o Garlic (minced)

- One-fourth tsp. of cumin (ground)

- Two cups of rotisserie chicken

- Four tsps. of lime juice

- One-eighth tsp. of each

  o Pepper

  o Salt

- Seven cups of tortilla chips

- Eight ounces of pepper jack cheese (shredded)

- One-fourth cup of green onion (sliced)

- Half cup of cilantro (minced)

- One cup of sour cream

- Two tsps. of pickled jalapeno peppers (diced)

Method:

1. Sauté the pepper in a skillet with one tsp. of oil. Cook for three minutes. Keep aside.

2. Add garlic, beans, cumin, and oregano in the same skillet. Cook for three minutes.

3. Combine lime juice, chicken, pepper, and salt in a bowl. Grease a baking dish with some oil.

4. Create a layer of tortilla chips with half of the chips. Layer with pepper mixture, chicken, bean mixture, onion, cheese, and cilantro. Repeat for the remaining layers.

5. Bake for twenty minutes.

6. Serve hot with pickled jalapenos and sour cream.

Santa Fe Salad (The Cheesecake Factory)

Total Prep & Cooking Time: One hour and twenty minutes

Yields: Six servings

Nutrition Facts: Calories: 970.3 | Protein: 48.7g | Carbs: 64.7g | Fat: 57.2g | Fiber: 12.1g

Ingredients

- Four breasts of chicken
- Half cup of teriyaki sauce

For the dressing:

- One-fourth cup of cilantro (chopped)
- Two tbsps. of peanut butter
- One tbsp. of each
    - Red wine vinegar
    - Lime juice
    - Brown sugar
- Three garlic cloves (minced)
- One tsp. of each
    - Sesame oil

       o   Lime zest

       o   Black pepper (ground)

- Half cup of olive oil

- Three corn tortillas

For the salad:

- One can of sweet corn (drained)

- One can of black beans (drained)

- One head of romaine lettuce

- Two cups of Monterey cheese

Method:

1. Mix chicken breasts with teriyaki sauce in a bowl. Refrigerate for one hour.

2. Mix peanut butter, cilantro, lime juice, red wine vinegar, garlic, brown sugar, lime zest, and sesame oil in a blender. Add the olive oil along with peppers. Blend again.

3. Preheat your oven at one-hundred and seventy-five degrees Celsius. Spread the tortillas on a baking tray; sprinkle two tsps. of oil. Bake for ten minutes. Cut into thin strips.

4. Heat two tbsps. of oil in a large skillet. Add the beasts of chicken and cook for ten

minutes on each side. Slice the cooked chicken breast into strips.

5. Mix black beans, corn, and lettuce in a mixing bowl. Add chicken, strips of tortilla, and cheese.

6. Add the dressing and toss.

Tex Mex Egg Rolls (The Cheesecake Factory)

Total Prep & Cooking Time: Forty minutes

Yields: Twenty-four servings

Nutrition Facts: Calories: 143.2 | Protein: 6.8g | Carbs: 14.6g | Fat: 7.3g | Fiber: 1.5g

Ingredients

- One tbsp. of canola oil
- Two cups of cooked chicken breast (diced)
- Half yellow onion (diced)
- One garlic clove (minced)
- One tsp. of each
  - Chili powder
  - Cumin
- Half tsp. of kosher salt
- One cup of each
  - Corn
  - Black beans
- One green bell pepper (diced)
- One tomato (diced)

- Half cup of cheddar cheese (shredded)

- Two tbsps. of cilantro (chopped)

- Twenty-four egg roll wrappers

- Oil (for frying)

For the dipping sauce:

- Eight ounces of cream cheese

- One-fourth cup of sour cream

- One bunch of cilantro

- Half avocado

Method:

1. Add oil in a skillet. Add onion, garlic, chicken, chili powder, cumin, and salt. Cook for one minute. Keep aside.

2. Add black beans, corn, tomato, bell pepper, cilantro, and cheddar cheese to the chicken mixture. Mix well.

3. Arrange the egg roll wrappers on a working surface. Add three tbsps. of the filling mixture in the center of each wrapper. Roll the wrappers and seal the ends.

4. Heat canola oil in a large pan. Add the rolls and cook for four minutes.

5. Combine the listed ingredients for the dipping sauce in a small bowl.

6. Serve the rolls hot with dipping sauce by the side.

Hot Wings (Pluckers Wing Bar)

Total Prep & Cooking Time: Forty minutes

Yields: Four servings

Nutrition Facts: Calories: 806.3 | Protein: 32.4g | Carbs: 3.3g | Fat: 80.6g | Fiber: 2.1g

Ingredients

- Three pounds of chicken wings

- Two cups of hot sauce

- Half cup of butter

- Two tsps. of black pepper (ground)

- Two jalapenos (sliced)

- One and a half tsp. of vinegar

- Oil (to fry)

Method:

1. Heat the oil in a deep pan. Add the chicken wings. Deep-fry the chicken wings for ten minutes.

2. Combine butter, hot sauce, jalapeno, vinegar, and black pepper in a bowl. Mix well.

3. Add the fried wings in a large mixing bowl; pour the sauce all over the wings. Toss for coating the wings in the sauce.

4. Serve hot.

Blooming Onion (Outback Steakhouse)

Total Prep & Cooking Time: Forty minutes

Yields: Four servings

Nutrition Facts: Calories: 727.6 | Protein: 7.5g | Carbs: 32.4g | Fat: 71.6g | Fiber: 2.1g

Ingredients

- Half cup of mayonnaise

- Three-fourth tbsp. of ketchup

- Two tbsps. of horseradish sauce

- One-fourth tsp. of each

  - Paprika

  - Salt

- One tsp. of each

  - Black pepper (black)

  - Cayenne pepper

- One large egg

- One cup of milk

- Half cup of flour

- One and a half tsp. of salt

- Two tsps. of each

  - Cayenne pepper

  - Black pepper (ground)

  - Thyme (dried)

  - Oregano (dried)

  - Garlic powder

- One-eighth tsp. of cumin (ground)

- One large onion

- Two cups of oil (to fry)

Method:

1. Combine horseradish sauce, mayonnaise, ketchup, one-fourth tsp. of salt, paprika, one pinch of black pepper, and half tsp. of cayenne pepper. Mix well.

2. Combine milk with egg.

3. Combine salt, flour, cayenne pepper, garlic powder, black pepper, oregano, cumin, and thyme in another bowl.

4. For preparing the onion, cut one-inch from the top and bottom. Cut out one-inch of core from the center of the onion. Use a sharp knife for slicing down the middle of the onion. Slice up to three-

fourth of the length. Turn the onion ninety degrees and slice it again. Continue doing this until you have sixteen sections in total. Use your hand to spread the onion petals.

5. Dip the prepared onion in the mixture of egg and milk. Coat in the mixture of flour. Repeat again.

6. Let the coated onion rest in the refrigerator for fifteen minutes.

7. Heat oil in a deep pan. Fry the onion for ten minutes.

8. Drain excess oil with the help of paper towels.

9. Pour the dipping sauce in a small bowl.

10. Serve the onion with dipping sauce by the side.

Fried Mushrooms (Outback Steakhouse)

Total Prep & Cooking Time: Forty minutes

Yields: Four servings

Nutrition Facts: Calories: 189.6 | Protein: 7.6g | Carbs: 32.3g| Fat: 4.4g | Fiber: 2.6g

Ingredients

- Eight ounces of whole mushrooms

- Half cup of flour

- Oil (to fry)

- Half tsp. of each

  o Salt

  o Black pepper (ground)

- One-fourth tsp. of each

  o Paprika

  o Dry mustard

- One cup of buttermilk

- One tsp. of cayenne pepper

Method:

1. Start by washing the mushrooms. Remove the stems.

2. Combine salt, flour, cayenne pepper, black pepper, paprika, and mustard in a bowl.

3. Pour the buttermilk in another bowl.

4. Dip the mushrooms in buttermilk and coat them in the mixture of flour.

5. Heat oil in a frying pan. Add the coated mushrooms. Fry for three minutes.

6. Serve hot.

Gorgonzola Crescent (Red Lobster)

Total Prep & Cooking Time: Two hours and forty minutes

Yields: Four servings

Nutrition Facts: Calories: 810.3 | Protein: 24.3g | Carbs: 89.6g| Fat: 37.2g | Fiber: 6.9g

Ingredients

- Five-hundred grams of flour

- Two-hundred grams of gorgonzola cheese

- Thirty grams of yeast

- Half cup of water

- One-third cup of lard

- One-fourth cup of butter

- Half tsp. of salt

Method:

1. Start by placing the flour on a flat working surface. Make a small well in the center. Add yeast, cheese, lard, water, butter, and salt in the prepared well.

2. Knead the dough properly. Let the dough sit for one hour.

3. Use a rolling pin for rolling out the dough into a thickness of one inch. Cut the dough into squares.

4. Brush the cutout dough with egg.

5. Arrange the squares on a baking tray. Let them rise for thirty minutes.

6. Bake for thirty minutes.

The O-Ring Shorty (Red Robin)

Total Prep & Cooking Time: Twenty-five minutes

Yields: Four servings

Nutrition Facts: Calories: 156.3 | Protein: 4.6g | Carbs: 13.6g| Fat: 8.6g | Fiber: 1.3g

Ingredients

- One large onion
- Half cup of flour
- Half tsp. of baking powder
- One tsp. of salt
- One large egg
- One cup of milk
- One and a half cup of bread crumbs
- Oil (to fry)
- One-third tsp. of seasoned salt

Method:

1. Cut the onion into slices of one-fourth inch. Separate the slices into rings.

2. Combine salt, baking powder, and flour in a bowl.

3. Whisk milk and egg in a bowl.

4. Arrange the bread crumbs in a flat dish.

5. Coat the onion rings in the mixture of flour. Dip the rings in the egg mixture and then coat in bread crumbs.

6. Heat the oil in a pan. Fry the onion rings for thirty seconds.

7. Toss with seasoned salt.

CHAPTER 3:
APPETIZER RECIPES

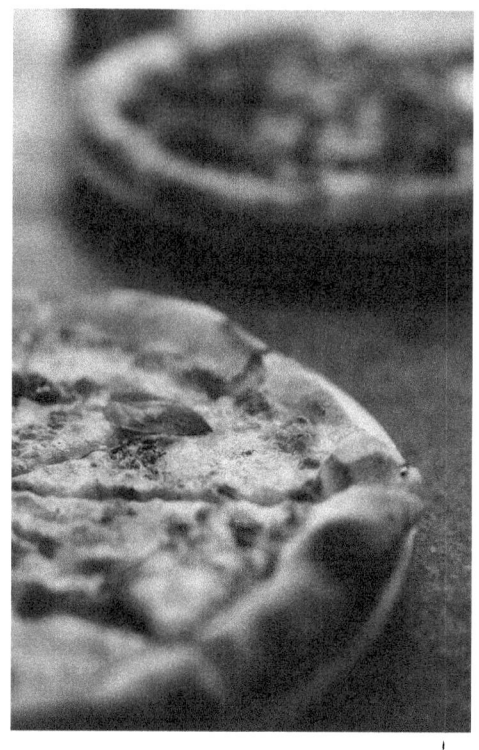

Mini Pizza (Red Lobster)

Total Prep & Cooking Time: Fifty minutes

Yields: Four servings

Nutrition Facts: Calories: 305.6 | Protein: 17.5g | Carbs: 20.4g| Fat: 14.6g | Fiber: 2.6g

Ingredients

- One shortcrust pastry

- One onion (chopped)

- One can of mushrooms

- Four-hundred grams of tomato pulp

- Salt (for seasoning)

- One tsp. of black pepper (ground)

- One can of anchovies

- Half cup of mozzarella cheese (grated)

Method:

1. Preheat your oven at two-hundred degrees Celsius.

2. Roll out the pastry dough. Cut out circles from the dough. You can use a pastry cutter.

3. Arrange the circles on a baking sheet.

4. Heat olive oil in a pan. Add mushrooms, onion, salt, pepper, and tomato pulp. Cook for five minutes.

5. Add the tomato mixture on the circles.

6. Add one piece of anchovy on each pizza circle and top with mozzarella.

7. Bake for twenty minutes.

8. Serve hot.

Sesame Pork (Red Lobster)

Total Prep & Cooking Time: Two hours and thirty minutes

Yields: Six servings

Nutrition Facts: Calories: 154.6 | Protein: 18.3g | Carbs: 2.6g| Fat: 10.9g | Fiber: 0.6g

Ingredients

- Two pounds of pork tenderloin

- Half cup of sherry (dry)

- One tbsp. of soy sauce

- One-third cup of each

    o Honey

    o Sesame seeds

    o Soy sauce

- One and a half tbsp. of each

    o Sherry (dry)

    o Sesame oil

- One garlic clove (minced)

- Half tsp. of ginger root (grated)

- One green onion (chopped)

Method:

1. Combine soy sauce along with sherry in a large bowl; add the tenderloin. Marinate the pork for two hours.

2. Spread the honey on a shallow dish. Arrange the sesame seeds on another dish.

3. Roll the marinated pork in honey and then coat in sesame seeds.

4. Roast in the oven for twenty minutes.

5. Slice the pork tenderloin.

6. Combine the remaining ingredients for preparing the dipping sauce.

7. Serve the pork slices hot with dipping sauce by the side.

Onion Soup (TGI Friday's)

Total Prep & Cooking Time: Two hours and forty minutes

Yields: Twelve servings

Nutrition Facts: Calories: 170.3 | Protein: 6.3g | Carbs: 15.6g| Fat: 9.2g | Fiber: 1.6g

Ingredients

- Five tbsps. of olive oil

- One tbsp. of butter

- Eight cups of onions (sliced)

- Three cloves of garlic (minced)

- Half cup of port wine

- Two cans of beef stock

- Half tsp. of pepper

- One-fourth tsp. of salt

- Twenty-four slices of baguette

- Two cloves of garlic (halved)

- Three-fourth cup of Swiss cheese (shredded)

Method:

1. Take an iron skillet and add butter along with two tbsps. of oil. Add the onions and cook for ten minutes. Add garlic and cook on low for thirty minutes.

2. Add the wine and boil the mixture; add beef stock, salt, and pepper. Reduce the flame. Simmer for one hour.

3. Preheat your oven at two-hundred degrees Celsius. Place the slices of baguette in the oven and brush with oil on both sides. Bake for three minutes.

4. Rub the baguette toasts with halves of garlic.

5. Place the baguette slices in soup bowls; pour soup from the top. Add the cheese. Broil for about four minutes.

6. Serve hot.

BBQ Chicken Salad (TGI Friday's)

Total Prep & Cooking Time: Three hours and forty minutes

Yields: Six servings

Nutrition Facts: Calories: 568.7 | Protein: 32.9g | Carbs: 45.6g| Fat: 24.6g | Fiber: 6.9g

Ingredients

- One bottle of barbecue sauce

- Two tbsps. of brown sugar

- Half tsp. of garlic powder

- One-fourth tsp. of paprika

- One pound of chicken breast

- Twelve romaine lettuce heads (chopped)

- Two avocados (chopped)

- Three plum tomatoes (chopped)

- Two carrots (sliced)

- One red pepper (chopped)

- Three large eggs (hard-boiled, chopped)

- Six strips of bacon (cooked, crumbled)

- One and a half cup of cheddar cheese (shredded)

- Salad dressing (any)

Method:

1. Grease a slow cooker with some oil. Add brown sugar, barbecue sauce, paprika, and garlic powder. Reserve half cup of sauce. Add the chicken breast. Cook the chicken for three hours.

2. Cut the chicken in bite-size pieces.

3. Toss the chicken pieces in the reserved sauce.

4. Arrange lettuce on a salad plate. Add avocado, chicken, eggs, vegetables, cheese, and bacon.

5. Serve by drizzling the dressing from the top.

Angry Alfredo (Olive Garden)

Total Prep & Cooking Time: Forty minutes

Yields: Four servings

Nutrition Facts: Calories: 585.6 | Protein: 20.3g | Carbs: 2.9g| Fat: 55.6g | Fiber: 1.6g

Ingredients

For the sauce:

- Four ounces of butter
- One cup of heavy cream
- Half cup of parmesan cheese (grated)
- Half tsp. of garlic powder
- One-fourth tsp. of red pepper flakes

For the chicken:

- Eight ounces of chicken breast
- Pepper and salt (for seasoning)
- One tbsp. of olive oil
- Half cup of mozzarella cheese

Method:

1. Take a medium-sized saucepan and add butter in it; add the cream along with the cheese. Simmer the mixture and add pepper flakes. Stir in the garlic powder and simmer for one minute.

2. Season the breast of chicken with pepper and salt.

3. Take an iron skillet and add olive oil in it. Add the chicken breast. Cook the chicken for seven minutes on each side.

4. Preheat the oven at broil setting.

5. Slice the chicken breast into small bite-size pieces. Mix the chicken pieces with the sauce.

6. Pour the chicken mixture into a large casserole dish. Top the chicken with mozzarella cheese.

7. Broil for five minutes.

8. Serve hot.

Grilled Chicken Flatbread (Olive Garden)

Total Prep & Cooking Time: Forty-five minutes

Yields: Four servings

Nutrition Facts: Calories: 441.3 | Protein: 21.6g | Carbs: 52.3g| Fat: 13.5g | Fiber: 2.6g

Ingredients

- Twelve ounces of flatbread

- Half pound of chicken breast

- One cup of alfredo sauce

- One red pepper (grilled)

- One-fourth cup of each

    o Basil (chopped)

    o Mozzarella cheese (shredded)

- One clove of garlic

Method:

1. Season the chicken with pepper and salt.

2. Heat a skillet and add some oil in it. Add the chicken. Cook for six minutes on each side.

3. Slice the chicken into small slices.

4. Preheat your oven at one-hundred and fifty degrees Celsius.

5. Cut the garlic clove in half. Rub it over the flatbreads.

6. Arrange the cooked chicken on the flatbreads. Add alfredo sauce and top with grilled pepper and cheese.

7. Bake for eight minutes.

8. Sprinkle basil from the top. Serve hot.

Fried Pickle Nickels (Red Robin)

Total Prep & Cooking Time: Twenty minutes

Yields: Four servings

Nutrition Facts: Calories: 95.6 | Protein: 1.2g | Carbs: 8.7g| Fat: 5.6g | Fiber: 1.6g

Ingredients

- Thirty-two ounces of dill pickles (whole)

- One cup of buttermilk

- Two tbsps. of hot sauce

- One cup of each

  - Cornmeal

  - Flour

- Two and a half tbsp. of garlic salt

- One and a half tbsp. of paprika

- One tbsp. of cayenne pepper

- One tsp. of pepper

- Oil (to fry)

Method:

1. Drain the pickles and discard the liquid. Use a knife for cutting the pickles into slices of half-inch. Use paper towels for drying the pickles.

2. Mix hot sauce with buttermilk in a bowl.

3. Take another shallow bowl and combine cornmeal, flour, paprika, garlic salt, pepper, and cayenne pepper.

4. Start dipping the slices of pickle in the buttermilk mixture and then coat them in the mixture of flour.

5. Heat oil in a deep pan. Add the pickles and deep fry them for three minutes.

6. Serve hot.

Arctic Cod Fish and Chips (Red Robin)

Total Prep & Cooking Time: One hour and twenty minutes

Yields: Four servings

Nutrition Facts: Calories: 465.6 | Protein: 21.6g | Carbs: 39.6g| Fat: 23.6g | Fiber: 5.3g

Ingredients

- One-third cup of mayonnaise

- Two tbsps. of dill pickle (chopped)

- Two tsps. of lemon zest

For the fish and chips:

- One pound of baking potatoes

- Two tsps. of olive oil

- Three-fourth tsp. of kosher salt

- Half tsp. of ground black pepper

- One-third cup of panko bread crumbs

- One-fourth cup of seasoned bread crumbs

- Four fillets of cod

- Two tbsps. of each

- ○ Parmesan cheese (grated)

- ○ Mayonnaise

- One tsp. of parsley (chopped)

Method:

1. For the dipping sauce, combine mayonnaise, lemon zest, and pickle. Mix well and refrigerate.

2. Preheat your oven at two hundred degrees Celsius.

3. Cut the potatoes into wedges of one-inch lengthwise. Toss the potato wedges with oil, one-fourth tsp. of pepper, or half tsp. of salt.

4. Spread the potato wedges in a baking pan. Roast for forty minutes.

5. Take a small skillet and toast the bread crumbs. Keep aside.

6. Take the cod fillets and sprinkle with pepper and salt.

7. Spread mayonnaise on the fillets and dip in the mixture of bread crumbs.

8. Arrange the fillets in a greased baking dish. Bake for fifteen minutes.

9. Toss the wedges of potato with parsley and cheese.

10. Serve the fish fillets with dipping sauce and chips.

Chili Cheese Fries (Red Robin)

Total Prep & Cooking Time: Six hours and twenty minutes

Yields: Sixteen servings

Nutrition Facts: Calories: 371.3 | Protein: 18.9g | Carbs: 31.3g| Fat: 15.6g | Fiber: 5.3g

Ingredients

- One medium-sized onion (chopped)

- One carrot (chopped)

- Two pounds of beef stew meat (cut in pieces of half-inch)

- Three tbsps. of flour

- Two tbsps. of canola oil

- One can of diced tomatoes

- One ounce of chili seasoning mix

- Fifteen ounces of pinto beans (rinsed)

- One green pepper (chopped)

- One jalapeno pepper (chopped)

- Thirty-two ounces of French-fried potatoes

- Two cups of cheddar cheese (shredded)

Method:

1. Add carrot and onion in a slow cooker.

2. Toss the beef with two tbsps. of flour.

3. Take a skillet. Add oil in it. Add the beef and cook until browned.

4. Pour the cooked beef in the slow cooker.

5. Drain the tomatoes and reserve the liquid.

6. In a small mixing ball, combine drained liquid, remaining flour, and chili seasoning. Mix well.

7. Pour the flour mixture over the beef; add the beans, peppers, and tomatoes. Stir for combining.

8. Cook for six hours.

9. Cook the potatoes in accordance with the instructions on the package.

10. Arrange the fries on a plate. Top with the beef and chili mixture. Add cheese from the top.

11. Serve hot.

Cheese Fries (Texas Roadhouse)

Total Prep & Cooking Time: Thirty minutes

Yields: Four servings

Nutrition Facts: Calories: 259.6 | Protein: 9.2g | Carbs: 23.6g| Fat: 13.5g | Fiber: 2.2g

Ingredients

- Four cups of waffle-cut fries (frozen)

- Two tsps. of steak seasoning

- One cup of cheddar cheese (shredded)

- Two tbsps. of each

  o   Bacon bits

  o   Green onion (chopped)

Method:

1. Add the waffle fries in a baking pan greased with some oil. Bake for twenty minutes at one-hundred and seventy-five degrees Celsius.

2. Sprinkle the steak seasoning over the fries; add the remaining ingredients. Toss for combining.

3. Bake for three minutes.

4. Serve hot.

Avo-Cobb-O Salad (Red Robin)

Total Prep & Cooking Time: Forty minutes

Yields: Six servings

Nutrition Facts: Calories: 570.2 | Protein: 18.2g | Carbs: 9.6g| Fat: 48.3g | Fiber: 5.3g

Ingredients

- One-fourth cup of red wine vinegar

- Two tsps. of salt

- One tsp. lemon juice

- One garlic clove(minced)

- Three-fourth tsp. of ground pepper

- One-third tsp. of Worcestershire sauce

- One-fourth tsp. of each

    o   Mustard (ground)

    o   Sugar

- One-third cup of canola oil

- Half cup of olive oil

For the salad:

- Four cups of romaine (torn)

- Two cups of curly endive (torn)

- One bunch of watercress (trimmed)

- Two chicken breasts (cooked, chopped)

- Two tomatoes (chopped)

- One avocado (chopped)

- Three boiled eggs (chopped)

- Half cup of blue cheese (crumbled)

- Six strips of bacon (cooked, crumbled)

- Two tbsps. of chives (minced)

Method:

1. Combine the first eight listed ingredients in a high power blender. Add olive oil and canola oil. Blend well.

2. Combine all the listed salad ingredients in a large bowl.

3. Pour the dressing over the salad. Toss to combine.

Rattlesnake Bites (Texas Roadhouse)

Total Prep & Cooking Time: Forty-five minutes

Yields: Six servings

Nutrition Facts: Calories: 61.3 | Protein: 2.6g | Carbs: 9.6g| Fat: 1.6g | Fiber: 0.6g

Ingredients

- Two eight ounces blocks of pepper jack cheese (shredded)

- Half cup of flour

- Three jalapenos (diced)

- One large egg

- Two cups of bread crumbs

- One tsp. of cayenne pepper

- Half tsp. of paprika

- One-third tsp. of garlic powder

- Oil (to fry)

Method:

1. Combine jalapenos and cheese in a large bowl.

2. Use your hands to shape the mixture of cheese into balls of one-inch.

3. Refrigerate the cheese balls for thirty minutes.

4. Add the flour in a bowl.

5. Mix milk and eggs in another bowl.

6. Combine the seasonings and bread crumbs in a bowl.

7. Dip the cheese balls in the mixture of flour and then in the milk mixture

8. Roll the balls in the mixture of bread crumbs.

9. Fry the cheese balls in hot oil for four minutes.

10. Serve hot.

CHAPTER 4:
SOUP RECIPES

Zuppa Toscana (Olive garden)

Total Prep & Cooking Time: Forty-five minutes

Yields: Six servings

Nutrition Facts: Calories: 401.3 | Protein: 14.5g | Carbs: 30.2g| Fat: 23.4g | Fiber: 3.2g

Ingredients

- One pound of Italian ground sausage (spicy)

- Four tbsps. of water

- Half a white onion (diced)

- One tbsp. of garlic (minced)

- Six cups of chicken stock

- Two cups of water

- Five yellow potatoes (cut in one-inch piece)

- Three tsps. of salt

- One tsp. of black pepper (ground)

- Two cups of heavy cream

- Four cups of kale (chopped)

- Four tbsps. of parmesan cheese (grated)

- Bacon (chopped, for garnishing)

Method:

1. Take a large pot and sauté the sausage meat for six minutes. Keep aside.

2. Add butter in the same pot. Sauté the onions and add garlic. Cook for three minutes.

3. Add the chicken stock along with water, salt, potatoes, and pepper. Boil the mixture. Keep boiling until the potatoes are soft.

4. Add heavy cream and kale. Stir for mixing.

5. Add the sausage meat and simmer for five minutes.

6. Garnish with cheese and bacon.

7. Serve hot.

Minestrone Soup (Olive Garden)

Total Prep & Cooking Time: Forty-five minutes

Yields: Six servings

Nutrition Facts: Calories: 302.3 | Protein: 14.9g | Carbs: 47.9g| Fat: 5.1g | Fiber: 11.3g

Ingredients

- Two tbsps. of olive oil

- Three-fourth cup of onion (diced)

- Half cup of each

    o Carrots (sliced)

    o Celery (sliced)

    o Shell pasta

    o Green beans (cut, frozen)

- Two tsps. of garlic (minced)

- One zucchini (sliced)

- Pepper and salt (to taste)

- One can of diced tomatoes

- Four cups of vegetable stock

- One-fourth cup of tomato paste

- Two and a half tsp. of Italian seasoning

- One can of white beans (small, rinsed)

- One and a half can of kidney beans (rinsed)

- Two cups of each

  o Parsley (chopped)

  o Spinach leaves

Method:

1. Heat oil in a large pot. Add celery, onion, zucchini, and carrots. Cook for five minutes. Add the minced garlic. Cook for thirty seconds.

2. Add pepper and salt.

3. Add vegetable stock, tomatoes, Italian seasoning, and tomato paste. Simmer the mixture; add kidney beans, white beans, green beans, and pasta. Simmer for fifteen minutes.

4. Add spinach leaves. Cook for three minutes.

5. Add parsley.

6. Serve hot.

Hot And Sour Soup (Panda Express)

Total Prep & Cooking Time: Thirty minutes

Yields: Six servings

Nutrition Facts: Calories: 104.6 | Protein: 9.1g | Carbs: 6.5g| Fat: 3.7g | Fiber: 0.7g

Ingredients

- Six cups of chicken stock

- Six tbsps. of soy sauce

- Three-fourth cup of button mushrooms (sliced)

- Two tsps. of chili garlic sauce

- Half tsp. of white pepper (ground)

- Three tbsps. of each

    o Cold water

    o Cornstarch

- One large egg (beaten)

- Six ounces of tofu (firm, cubed)

- Two green onions (chopped)

- One-third cup of white vinegar

- Three-fourth tsp. of sesame oil

Method:

1. Simmer the chicken stock in a saucepan.

2. Add button mushrooms, soy sauce, white pepper, and chili garlic sauce. Simmer the mixture for five minutes.

3. Mix three tbsps. of cornstarch with two tbsps. of water.

4. Add the cornstarch mixture in the saucepan. Simmer for four minutes.

5. Add the egg and stir the soup.

6. Add the cubes of tofu and the green onions.

7. Remove the soup from heat.

8. Add sesame oil and vinegar.

9. Stir the soup.

10. Serve hot.

Veggie Soup (Cracker Barrel)

Total Prep & Cooking Time: Two hours

Yields: Eight servings

Nutrition Facts: Calories: 170.3 | Protein: 8.6g | Carbs: 23.5g| Fat: 4.1g | Fiber: 5.6g

Ingredients

- Five cups of vegetable stock

- Five cubes of beef bouillon

- Three cans of diced tomatoes

- Two stalks of celery (sliced)

- One can of green beans

- Twenty ounces of corn (frozen)

- Fifteen ounces of peas (frozen)

- Ten ounces of baby limas (frozen)

- Four cups of water

- One package of seasoning blend (bell pepper, onion, celery)

- Six ounces of beef stock

- Two potatoes (cubed)

- Pepper and salt (for seasoning)

Method:

1. Add all the listed ingredients in a large pot. Stir for combining.

2. Lower the flame and cover the pot. Simmer for one hour.

3. Serve hot.

Chicken Tortilla Soup (Red Robin)

Total Prep & Cooking Time: One hour and ten minutes

Yields: Eight servings

Nutrition Facts: Calories: 160.3 | Protein: 24.2g | Carbs: 11.2g| Fat: 17.1g | Fiber: 2.9g

Ingredients

- Eight ounces of each
    - Celery (sliced)
    - Carrots (diced)
    - Onions (diced)
- Half tsp. of garlic powder
- One-eighth tsp. of salt
- One-fourth tsp. of pepper
- One tbsp. of corn oil
- Four cans of chicken stock
- One can of tomatoes (diced)
- Ten ounces of chilies and tomato mix (diced)
- One ounce of taco seasoning

- Ten corn tortillas (cut in one-inch pieces)

- Twelve ounces of chicken (diced, poached)

- One cup of milk

- Eight ounces of Monterey jack cheese

Method:

1. Sauté onions, carrots, garlic, and celery in corn oil. Add pepper and salt.

2. Add the chicken stock and boil the mixture.

3. Add taco seasoning, tomatoes, chili and tomato mix, and chicken.

4. Add the tortillas.

5. Boil the mixture for forty minutes.

6. Lower the flame and add the cheese. Simmer for ten minutes.

7. Add the milk and simmer for five minutes.

8. Garnish the soup with shredded cheese.

9. Serve hot.

Country Potato Soup (McAlister's Deli)

Total Prep & Cooking Time: Forty-five minutes

Yields: Eight servings

Nutrition Facts: Calories: 218.2 | Protein: 6.6g | Carbs: 23.5g| Fat: 11.9g | Fiber: 2.2g

Ingredients

- Six strips of bacon (diced)
- Three cups of potatoes (cubed)
- One carrot (grated)
- Half cup of onion (chopped)
- One tbsp. of parsley flakes (dried)
- Half tsp. of each
  - Pepper
  - Salt
  - Celery seed
- One can of chicken stock
- Three tbsps. of flour
- Three cups of milk
- Eight ounces of cheese (cubed)

- Two green onions (sliced)

Method:

1. Take a large saucepan. Heat oil in it.

2. Add bacon and cook for five minutes.

3. Add seasonings, chicken stock, and veggies. Boil the mixture.

4. Simmer for fifteen minutes.

5. Combine milk and flour in a bowl. Stir the milk mixture in the soup.

6. Boil the soup and stir for two minutes.

7. Add the cheese.

8. Boil for one minute.

9. Garnish with green onions.

10. Serve hot.

Southwest Chicken Soup (Chili's)

Total Prep & Cooking Time: Forty-five minutes

Yields: Eight servings

Nutrition Facts: Calories: 169.3 | Protein: 15.6g | Carbs: 11.6g| Fat: 7.6g | Fiber: 1.3g

Ingredients

- One pound of chicken breast

- One tsp. of garlic (minced)

- One cup of white onion (chopped)

- Half cup of celery (chopped)

- Two tbsps. of vegetable oil

- One tbsp. of tomato paste

- Two cups of chicken stock

- One and a half tsp. of chipotle peppers in adobo sauce

- One and a half cup of white hominy

- Four ounces of green chili (diced)

- One-third cup of tomatoes (diced)

- One tsp. of lime juice

- Tortilla strips (fried)

- Cheese (grated)

Method:

1. Add one tbsp. of oil in a large pot.

2. Season the chicken with salt.

3. Add the chicken to the pot. Cook for seven minutes.

4. Shred the chicken and keep aside.

5. Add one tbsp. of oil in the same pot. Add onion and garlic. Cook for two minutes and add celery.

6. Add the tomato paste along with chicken stock. Stir well.

7. Add hominy, chipotle peppers, diced tomatoes, green chilies, and cooked chicken. Add lime juice and boil for two minutes.

8. Garnish with cheese and tortilla strips.

9. Serve hot.

Chicken Noodle Soup (Noodles & Company)

Total Prep & Cooking Time: Forty-five minutes

Yields: Eight servings

Nutrition Facts: Calories: 187.6 | Protein: 20.1g | Carbs: 14.9g| Fat: 6.2g | Fiber: 3.6g

Ingredients

- One tbsp. of canola oil
- Two ribs of celery (chopped)
- Two carrots (chopped)
- One onion (chopped)
- Eight cups of chicken broth
- Half tsp. of basil (dried)
- One-fourth tsp. of pepper
- Three cups of egg noodles
- Four cups of rotisserie chicken (chopped)
- One and a half tbsp. of parsley (minced)

Method:

1. Heat oil in a large pot. Add carrots, celery, and onion. Cook for seven minutes.

2. Add chicken broth, pepper, and basil. Boil the mixture.

3. Add the noodles and cook for twelve minutes.

4. Add parsley and chicken. Simmer for two minutes.

5. Serve hot.

Broccoli Cheddar Soup (Panera Bread)

Total Prep & Cooking Time: One hour and five minutes

Yields: Eight servings

Nutrition Facts: Calories: 301.3 | Protein: 13.4g | Carbs: 9.7g| Fat: 21.6g | Fiber: 1.9g

Ingredients

- One tbsp. of butter

- Half onion (chopped)

- One-fourth cup of each

    o Butter (melted)

    o Flour

- Two cups of each

    o Chicken stock

    o Milk

- One and a half cup of broccoli florets (chopped)

- One cup of carrots (cut in matchsticks)

- One celery stalk (sliced)

- Two and a half cup of cheddar cheese (shredded)

- One pinch of black pepper and salt (for seasoning)

Method:

1. Add one tbsp. of butter in a large skillet. Add the onions and sauté for five minutes. Keep aside.

2. Combine flour and one-fourth cup of butter in a saucepan. Cook for four minutes.

3. Add milk in the mixture of flour. Pour in the chicken stock. Simmer for twenty minutes.

4. Add sautéed onions, carrots, broccoli, and celery. Simmer for twenty minutes.

5. Add cheddar cheese and stir well.

6. Season with pepper and salt.

7. Serve hot.

CHAPTER 5: CHICKEN, PORK, AND BEEF RECIPES

Tuscan Garlic Chicken (Olive Garden)

Total Prep & Cooking Time: Forty-five minutes

Yields: Four servings

Nutrition Facts: Calories: 910.3 | Protein: 51.2g | Carbs: 112.6g| Fat: 30.2g | Fiber: 7.6g

Ingredients

For the chicken:

- One cup of flour
- Half cup of bread crumbs
- One tbsp. of garlic powder
- Two tsps. of Italian seasoning
- One tsp. of sea salt
- Half tsp. of each
    - Basil (dried)
    - Black pepper (ground)
    - Oregano (dried)

- Three chicken breasts
- Two tbsps. of olive oil

For the pasta:

- One pound of fettuccine

For the sauce:

- Two tbsps. of butter
- Four garlic cloves (minced)
- One red bell pepper (cut in strips of two-inch)
- Half tsp. of sea salt
- One-fourth tsp. of paprika
- One-eighth tsp. of black pepper (ground)
- Two tbsps. of flour
- One cup of chicken stock
- Half cup of milk
- One-third cup of half and half
- Two cups of spinach (chopped)
- One and a half cup of parmesan cheese (grated)

Method:

1. Preheat your oven at two-hundred degrees Celsius. Line a baking tray with the use of parchment paper.

2. Combine bread crumbs, flour, garlic powder, salt, Italian seasoning, pepper, oregano, and basil. Coat the chicken breasts in the prepared mixture of flour.

3. Take a skillet; add oil in it. Place the chicken breasts in the pan. Sear for three minutes on each side.

4. Place the chicken on the baking sheet. Bake for twenty minutes.

5. Heat water in a deep and large pot. Cook the pasta in accordance with the instructions on the packet. Drain and keep aside.

6. Add butter in a skillet. Add bell pepper. Cook for four minutes. Add pepper, paprika, and salt for seasoning. Add the garlic. Cook for one minute.

7. Add flour and constantly for one minute; add milk, chicken stock, and half and half. Simmer the mixture and add the spinach. Cook for five minutes.

8. Add the cheese and stir. Add the cooked pasta and mix well

9. Serve the pasta in serving bowls and top it with chicken.

Pork Filettino (Olive Garden)

Total Prep & Cooking Time: Five hours

Yields: Four servings

Nutrition Facts: Calories: 609.1 | Protein: 61.3g | Carbs: 4.6g| Fat: 35.7g | Fiber: 0.9g

Ingredients

- Four pork tenderloins

- Eight tbsps. of olive oil (extra virgin)

- Four tbsps. of each:

  o Rosemary (chopped)

  o Garlic (minced)

- Two tbsps. of parsley (chopped)

- Half tsp. of black pepper (ground)

- One tsp. of salt

Method:

1. Sprinkle pepper and salt on all sides of the pork tenderloins.

2. Combine olive oil, garlic, rosemary, and parsley in a small bowl. Brush the pork tenderloins with this mixture.

3. Marinate the tenderloins for two hours.

4. Heat a grill.

5. Grill the pork tenderloins for three hours or until soft.

6. Serve hot.

Braised Beef And Tortellini (Olive Garden)

Total Prep & Cooking Time: Three hours and thirty minutes

Yields: Six servings

Nutrition Facts: Calories: 1106.3 | Protein: 64.7g | Carbs: 81.3g| Fat: 56.8g | Fiber: 6.9g

Ingredients

- Four pounds of short ribs

- One tsp. of salt

- Half tsp. of black pepper (ground)

- Three tbsps. of olive oil (extra virgin)

- One cup of onion (diced)

- One-fourth cup of basil (chopped)

- One and a half cup of cooking wine

- Two cups of beef broth

- Half cup of water

- One bay leaf

- Two caps of portabella mushrooms

- Two tomatoes (each cut in four pieces)

- One tbsp. of balsamic vinegar

- Two tbsps. of butter

- Three and a half tbsp. of flour

- One-third cup of heavy cream

- Twenty ounces of cheese-filled tortellini

Method:

1. Preheat your oven at one-hundred and seventy degrees Celsius.

2. Add pepper and salt on all sides of the short ribs.

3. Heat oil in an iron skillet.

4. Add the ribs. Sear for three minutes on all sides. Keep aside. Reserve the beef fat.

5. Add onions in the skillet; cook for three minutes and add the basil. Add the wine and stir.

6. Add bay leaf and water. Cook for one minute.

7. Place the beef ribs back in the skillet.

8. Place the skillet in the oven. Let the beef ribs braise for two hours.

9. Take a pan and add the reserved beef fat. Add the mushroom caps and sauté for five minutes.

10. Add the tomatoes; stir in the vinegar. Keep aside.

11. Cook the tortellini by following the instructions on the packet. Drain and keep aside.

12. Take out the skillet from the oven. Place the beef ribs on a cutting board and remove the bones. Use a knife for slicing the beef.

13. Melt butter in a pan. Add the flour; add the beef juice. Stir well to combine.

14. Add the cream and mix again. Add the beef, tomatoes, and mushrooms.

15. Divide the tortellini among serving plates. Top with braised beef.

Alice Springs Chicken (Outback Steakhouse)

Total Prep & Cooking Time: One hour and five minutes

Yields: Two servings

Nutrition Facts: Calories: 879.6 | Protein: 71.3g | Carbs: 30.9g| Fat: 51.2g | Fiber: 4.6g

Ingredients

- Four chicken breasts
- Half cup of mustard
- Six bacon slices
- One-third cup of honey
- Two tsps. of onion flakes (dried)
- One cup of mushrooms (sliced)
- Two cups of jack cheese (shredded)
- One and a half cup of mayonnaise

Method:

1. Rub the chicken breasts with salt on all sides. Refrigerate for thirty minutes.

2. Heat a skillet and add the bacon slices. Cook until crisp. Keep aside.

3. Add the chicken breasts in the skillet. Cook for five minutes on all sides in the bacon grease. Transfer the chicken to a casserole dish.

4. Combine mustard, mayonnaise, onion flakes, and honey in a bowl.

5. Spread three-fourths of the mustard sauce over the chicken breasts. Layer with bacon, mushrooms, and cheese.

6. Bake for thirty minutes at one-hundred and seventy degrees Celsius.

7. Serve the cooked chicken with mustard honey sauce by the side.

Grilled Pork Chops (Outback Steakhouse)

Total Prep & Cooking Time: Fifty minutes

Yields: Two servings

Nutrition Facts: Calories: 410.6 | Protein: 47.9g | Carbs: 21.3g| Fat: 11.6g | Fiber: 0.6g

Ingredients

- Two pork loin chops (boneless, one-inch thickness)

- Two tsps. of black pepper (ground)

- Six tsps. of salt

- One and a half tsp. of olive oil

- Four tsps. of paprika

- One tsp. of each

  - Garlic powder

  - Onion powder

  - Cayenne pepper

- Half tsp. of each

  - Turmeric

  - Coriander

For the sauce:

- One-fourth cup of each

  - Honey

  - Orange marmalade

- Half tsp. of mustard (dry)

Method:

1. Dry the pork chops using paper towels.

2. Mix black pepper, salt, paprika, onion powder, garlic powder, cayenne pepper, coriander, and turmeric in a bowl.

3. Sprinkle the rub all over the chops; add olive oil. Rub it all over the pork chops.

4. Let the pork chops sit for ten minutes.

5. Heat a grill pan.

6. Add the pork chops and grill them for eight minutes on each side.

7. Turn the pork chops ninety degrees on each side for getting grill marks.

8. Mix honey, mustard, and orange marmalade in a bowl.

9. Serve the pork chops with the sauce by the side.

Beef Steak (Outback Steakhouse)

Total Prep & Cooking Time: Twenty minutes

Yields: Four servings

Nutrition Facts: Calories: 302.6 | Protein: 4.6g | Carbs: 6.7g| Fat: 5.2g | Fiber: 2.6g

Ingredients

- Four rib-eye steaks

- Six tsps. of salt

- Four tsps. of paprika

- Two tsps. of black pepper (ground)

- One tsp. of each

    o Garlic powder

    o Onion powder

    o Cayenne pepper

- Half tsp. of each

    o Turmeric

    o Coriander

Method:

1. Mix salt, paprika, black pepper, onion powder, garlic powder, cayenne pepper, coriander, and turmeric in a bowl.

2. Rub the spice mix all over the steaks.

3. Heat a frying pan on medium heat.

4. Sear the steaks for seven minutes on each side.

5. Serve hot.

Grilled Chicken Tenders (Cracker Barrel)

Total Prep & Cooking Time: One hour and ten minutes

Yields: Four servings

Nutrition Facts: Calories: 202.3 | Protein: 23.6g | Carbs: 3.1g| Fat: 9.3g | Fiber: 2.1g

Ingredients

- One pound of chicken breast tenders
- Half cup of Italian dressing
- One tsp. of lime juice
- Two tsps. of honey

Method:

1. Combine Italian dressing, honey, and lime juice in a bowl.

2. Pour the dressing mixture over the chicken. Mix well and marinate for one hour.

3. Take a non-stick pan. Heat it over medium flame. Add the chicken pieces and braise them until golden in color on all sides.

4. Serve hot.

Meatloaf (Cracker Barrel)

Total Prep & Cooking Time: One hour and five minutes

Yields: Eight servings

Nutrition Facts: Calories: 360.3 | Protein: 19.6g | Carbs: 23.9g| Fat: 18.6g | Fiber: 0.7g

Ingredients

- Two large eggs

- Two-third cup of milk

- Thirty-two Ritz crackers (crushed)

- Half cup of onion (chopped)

- Four ounces of cheddar cheese (shredded)

- One tsp. of salt

- One-fourth tsp. of pepper

- Two pounds of beef (ground)

- One-third cup of each
  - Brown sugar
  - Ketchup

- One and a half tsp. of mustard

Method:

1. Preheat your oven at one-hundred and seventy degrees Celsius.

2. Beat the eggs.

3. Add crackers and milk in a bowl; add the beaten eggs. Add cheese and onion. Mix well.

4. For seasoning, add pepper and salt. Add the ground beef and mix well.

5. Pour the beef mixture into a loaf tin.

6. Bake for forty minutes at one-hundred and fifty degrees Celsius.

7. Mix brown sugar, ketchup, and mustard in a bowl.

8. After thirty minutes of baking, spoon half of the ketchup mixture over the meatloaf and spread evenly. Bake for ten minutes.

9. Spoon the remaining ketchup mixture on the meatloaf and bake again for five minutes.

10. Use a knife for running along the edges of the loaf.

11. Place the loaf on a plate and slice it using a sharp knife.

12. Serve hot.

Shanghai Angus Steak (Panda Express)

Total Prep & Cooking Time: Thirty minutes

Yields: Two servings

Nutrition Facts: Calories: 375.6 | Protein: 27.6g | Carbs: 40.3g| Fat: 10.3g | Fiber: 3.6g

Ingredients

- One tbsp. of cornstarch
- One-fourth cup of each
  - Orange juice
  - Cold water
- One and a half tbsp. of soy sauce
- Half tsp. of sesame oil
- One pinch of red pepper flakes
- Half pound of beef sirloin steak (boneless, cut in thin strips)
- Two tsps. of canola oil
- One clove of garlic (minced)
- One cup of rice (cooked)
- Three cups of vegetable blend

Method:

1. Combine cornstarch, water, orange juice, soy sauce, red pepper flakes, and sesame oil in a bowl.

2. Add one tbsp. of oil in an iron skillet. Add the beef strips and stir-fry for four minutes. Keep aside.

3. Add the vegetable blend along with the garlic. Cook for three minutes.

4. Add the mixture of cornstarch and mix well.

5. Boil the mixture for two minutes.

6. Add the cooked beef and stir for mixing.

7. Serve hot with rice.

Broccoli Beef (Panda Express)

Total Prep & Cooking Time: Thirty minutes

Yields: Two servings

Nutrition Facts: Calories: 303.8 | Protein: 28.6g | Carbs: 19.5g| Fat: 11.4g | Fiber: 4.2g

Ingredients

- One tbsp. of cornstarch

- Half cup of beef stock

- One-fourth cup of sherry

- Two tbsps. of soy sauce

- One and a half tbsp. of brown sugar

- One clove of garlic (minced)

- One tsp. of ginger (minced)

- Two tsps. of canola oil

- Half pound of beef sirloin steak (cut in strips of half-inch)

- Two cups of broccoli florets

- Eight green onions (cut in pieces of one-inch)

Method:

1. Mix beef stock, cornstarch, sherry, soy sauce, ginger, garlic, and brown sugar in a bowl.

2. Heat one tsp. of oil in an iron skillet. Add the beef and stir-fry for three minutes. Keep aside.

3. Add the broccoli florets in the skillet. Add green onions and cook for five minutes. Add the mixture of cornstarch and boil for two minutes.

4. Add the cooked beef and mix well.

5. Serve hot.

CHAPTER 6: BURGER AND SANDWICH RECIPES

McChicken Sandwich (McDonald's)

Total Prep & Cooking Time: Two hours

Yields: Four servings

Nutrition Facts: Calories: 620.7 | Protein: 36.6g | Carbs: 54.5g| Fat: 27.8g | Fiber: 4.3g

Ingredients

- One large egg

- One cup of water

- Half cup of each

    o Flour

    o Dry tempura mix

- Two tbsps. of cornmeal

- Two tsps. of salt

- One tsp. of onion powder

- One-fourth tsp. of black pepper (ground)

- One-eighth tsp. of garlic powder

- Four fillets of chicken breast

- Four hamburger buns

- One and a half cup of iceberg lettuce

- Four tomato slices

For the sauce:

- One-fourth cup of mayonnaise

- One pinch of onion powder

Method:

1. Mix mayonnaise and onion powder in a bowl. Keep in the refrigerator.

2. Combine egg and water in a bowl. Mix well.

3. Mix tempura mix, flour, pepper, salt, garlic powder, and onion powder in a large bowl.

4. Dip the chicken fillets in the egg mixture and then coat in the tempura mixture.

5. Keep the chicken fillets in the refrigerator for half an hour.

6. Fry the chicken for twelve minutes.

7. Toast the hamburger buns.

8. Add the sauce on one side of the bun; add tomato slice and lettuce. Add the chicken patty. Top with the other half of the bun.

9. Serve immediately.

Egg McMuffins (McDonald's)

Total Prep & Cooking Time: Fifteen minutes

Yields: One serving

Nutrition Facts: Calories: 370 | Protein: 24.2g | Carbs: 26.7g| Fat: 18.9g | Fiber: 1.2g

Ingredients

- One large egg
- One English muffin
- One slice of bacon
- One large slice of cheddar cheese
- Cooking spray

Method:

1. Start by cutting the English muffin in half.
2. Toast the muffin in a pan.
3. Cook the egg in a small skillet.
4. Remove the egg and add the bacon slice. Cook for one minute.
5. Add the cheese slice at the base of the muffin. Add cooked egg and cheese.
6. Top with the other half of the muffin.
7. Serve immediately.

Egg Salad Sandwich (Starbucks)

Total Prep & Cooking Time: Twenty minutes

Yields: Two servings

Nutrition Facts: Calories: 303.8 | Protein: 16.5g | Carbs: 23.6g| Fat: 15.8g | Fiber: 4.4g

Ingredients

- Three boiled eggs

- One tbsp. of mayonnaise

- One tsp. of Dijon mustard

- One and a half tbsp. of green onion (diced)

- Pepper and salt (to taste)

- Four slices of wheat bread

- A handful of baby arugula

Method:

1. Start by peeling the boiled eggs. Chop them and keep the eggs in a bowl.

2. Add green onions, mustard, mayonnaise, pepper, and salt. Mix well.

3. Add arugula to one slice of the bread. Top with the egg mixture. Add another slice of bread.

4. Repeat for the other sandwich.

5. Serve immediately.

Backyard Burger (Bob Evans)

Total Prep & Cooking Time: Thirty minutes

Yields: Eight servings

Nutrition Facts: Calories: 414.5 | Protein: 23.4g | Carbs: 21.6g| Fat: 28.9g | Fiber: 1.1g

Ingredients

- One pound of sausage (ground)

- One and a half pounds of beef (ground)

- Two tbsps. of Worcestershire sauce

- Half cup of parmesan cheese (grated)

- One-third tsp. of black pepper (ground)

- Eight hamburger buns

- One bunch of lettuce

- One cup of sliced tomatoes

- One-third cup of sliced onions

Method:

1. Combine ground sausage, beef, Worcestershire sauce, black pepper, and cheese in a bowl. Mix well.

2. Form eight patties from the beef mixture.

3. Heat a grill pan. Add some oil in it. Grill the patties for fifteen minutes on each side.

4. Layer the buns with tomatoes, lettuce, beef patty, and onions.

5. Serve immediately.

Smokehouse Burger (Texas Roadhouse)

Total Prep & Cooking Time: Thirty minutes

Yields: Eight servings

Nutrition Facts: Calories: 879.3 | Protein: 31.6g | Carbs: 45.2g| Fat: 58.2g | Fiber: 3.3g

Ingredients

- Two pounds of beef (ground)

- Two cups of barbeque sauce

- Two tsps. of seasoned salt

- One and a half pounds of mushroom (sliced)

- One onion (cut in rings)

- Half cup of butter

- One-third cup of jack cheese

- Eight burger buns

Method:

1. Start by dividing the beef into eight equal parts. Roll them into balls and press for making patties.

2. Heat a grill pan. Add the patties and grill for fifteen minutes on each side.

3. Heat two tbsps. of butter in an iron skillet. Add onions and mushrooms. Add seasoned salt and cook for two minutes.

4. Heat the barbeque sauce in a saucepan.

5. Cut the burger buns in half.

6. Add the sauce to one half of the bun; add mushrooms, cheese, and onion. Add the cooked patty and top with the other half of the bun.

7. Add the burgers to a skillet and press with another skillet from the top. This will help in melting the cheese.

8. Serve immediately.

Lobster Roll (Red Lobster)

Total Prep & Cooking Time: Forty-five minutes

Yields: Four servings

Nutrition Facts: Calories: 222.3 | Protein: 27.3g | Carbs: 21.2g| Fat: 3.3g | Fiber: 1.6g

Ingredients

- Two tbsps. of sea salt

- Two cups of lobster meat (chopped in bite-size piece)

- Half cup of celery (chopped)

- Six tbsps. of Greek yogurt

- One tsp. of black pepper (ground)

- Four hotdog buns

Method:

1. Add water in a pot. Add salt in it. Add the lobster meat and boil for five minutes. Drain the water.

2. Mix lobster meat, Greek yogurt, and celery in a bowl.

3. Add pepper and salt.

4. Refrigerate for thirty minutes.

5. Add an equal amount of lobster mixture into each hotdog bun.

6. Serve immediately.

CHAPTER 7:
PASTA RECIPES

Chicken Alfredo (Olive Garden)

Total Prep & Cooking Time: Thirty minutes

Yields: Four servings

Nutrition Facts: Calories: 980.3 | Protein: 30.2g | Carbs: 64.3g| Fat: 78.3g | Fiber: 3.3g

Ingredients

- Twelve ounces of fettuccine pasta

- Two tbsps. of olive oil

- Three cups of butter

- Two chicken breasts

- One and a half tsp. of salt

- Two tsps. of pepper (ground)

- Three garlic cloves (chopped)

- Three tbsps. of flour

- Two cups of heavy cream

- Three-fourth cup of parmesan cheese (grated)

- Two and a half tbsp. of parsley (chopped)

Method:

1. Cook the pasta by following the instructions on the package.

2. Heat oil in an iron skillet. Add two tbsps. of butter. Cook the chicken breasts for seven minutes on each side. Season with pepper and salt.

3. Slice the chicken.

4. Heat remaining butter in a pan. Add salt, garlic, and pepper. Cook for one minute.

5. Add flour and whisk well.

6. Add the cream slowly.

7. Add half a cup of cheese. Mix well.

8. Place the pasta on serving plates. Top with sauce and chopped chicken. Garnish with cheese.

Shrimp Pasta (Red Lobster)

Total Prep & Cooking Time: Thirty minutes

Yields: Six servings

Nutrition Facts: Calories: 489.6 | Protein: 18.6g | Carbs: 30.6g| Fat: 28.6g | Fiber: 1.7g

Ingredients

- One-third cup of olive oil

- Three cloves of garlic (minced)

- One pound of shrimp (peeled)

- Two-third cup of clam juice

- One-fourth cup of white wine

- One cup of heavy cream

- Half cup of parmesan cheese (grated)

- One-fourth tsp. of each

    o Oregano

    o Basil (dried)

- Eight ounces of pasta (cooked)

Method:

1. Heat oil in an iron skillet. Add the garlic. Cook for one minute.

2. Add the shrimps. Cook for three minutes. Keep aside.

3. Add the clam juice in the skillet. Boil the juice. Add the white wine and simmer for three minutes.

4. Add the cream. Keep stirring.

5. Add cheese and shrimp. Cook for two minutes.

6. Add the remaining listed ingredients except for the cooked pasta.

7. Pour the shrimp sauce over the pasta. Stir to combine.

8. Garnish with cheese.

Mac And Cheese (Cracker Barrel)

Total Prep & Cooking Time: Forty-five minutes

Yields: Six servings

Nutrition Facts: Calories: 560.3 | Protein: 17.3g | Carbs: 21.7g| Fat: 41.4g | Fiber: 1.9g

Ingredients

- Two tbsps. of each

    o Flour

    o Butter

- One cup of chicken stock

- One and a half cup of cream (heavy)

- Two and a half cup of Colby cheese (shredded)

- Three cups of pasta (uncooked)

- One tsp. of salt

- One-eighth tsp. of black pepper (ground)

Method:

1. Boil four cups of water along with some salt in a pot. Add some salt. Cook the pasta. Drain the water.

2. Melt the butter in a pan. Add the flour for making a roux. Add the chicken stock and whisk well.

3. Add the cream along with the cheese. Cook until the cheese melts.

4. Add the uncooked pasta.

5. Pour the pasta mixture in a baking dish. Bake for ten minutes.

6. Serve hot.

Cajun Chicken Pasta (TGI Friday's)

Total Prep & Cooking Time: Fifty minutes

Yields: Four servings

Nutrition Facts: Calories: 589.3 | Protein: 21.6g | Carbs: 42.6g| Fat: 30.3g | Fiber: 3.3g

Ingredients

- Ten ounces of fettuccine pasta

- One chicken breast (cooked, sliced)

- One tbsp. of parmesan cheese (grated)

- One tsp. of parsley (chopped)

- Two tbsps. of olive oil

- One and a half tbsp. of garlic (minced)

- Half cup of each

    o Onion (chopped)

    o Green pepper (chopped)

    o Red pepper (chopped)

- One cup of chicken stock

- One-eighth tsp. of cayenne pepper

- Three-fourth tbsp. of cornstarch

- Three tbsps. of cold water

- Pepper and salt (for seasoning)

Method:

1. Cook the pasta. Keep aside.

2. Heat oil in a large pan. Add the garlic. Sauté for thirty seconds.

3. Add the onions and peppers. Cook for two minutes.

4. Add the stock and simmer; add cayenne pepper. Simmer for ten minutes.

5. Combine water and cornstarch in a bowl; add the cornstarch mixture to the sauce. Add pepper and salt for seasoning.

6. Add the pasta. Toss for combining.

7. Serve the pasta in serving dishes. Top with sliced chicken. Garnish with cheese.

Pasta Fagioli (Olive Garden)

Total Prep & Cooking Time: Forty-five minutes

Yields: Eight servings

Nutrition Facts: Calories: 360.3 | Protein: 27.3g | Carbs: 42.5g| Fat: 3.4g | Fiber: 12.6g

Ingredients

- One pound of beef (ground)

- One yellow onion (diced)

- Four cloves of garlic (minced)

- Three carrots (diced)

- Two stalks of celery (diced)

- One can of kidney beans (drained)

- Fifteen ounces of cannellini beans (drained)

- Two cans of tomato sauce

- Half can of tomatoes (diced)

- Three cups of chicken stock

- One tsp. of each
    - Thyme leaves (dried)
    - Oregano (dried)

- Pepper and salt (for seasoning)

- Parmesan cheese (grated)

- One cup of ditalini pasta

Method:

1. Heat oil in an iron skillet. Add the beef. Cook for two minutes.

2. Add minced garlic, onion, celery, and carrots. Add pepper and salt. Cook for five minutes.

3. Add tomato sauce, cannellini beans, kidney beans, chicken stock, diced tomatoes, thyme, and oregano. Cook for five minutes.

4. Add the pasta when the liquid starts boiling.

5. Cook for ten minutes.

6. Garnish with cheese.

CHAPTER 8: JUICE AND DESSERT RECIPES

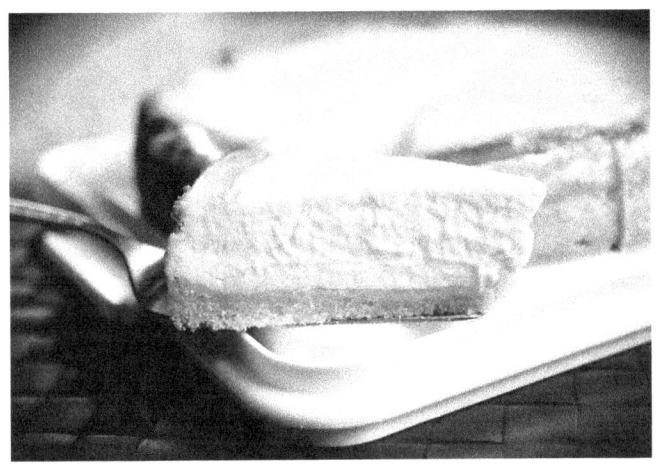

Choco Chip Cheesecake (The Cheesecake Factory)

Total Prep & Cooking Time: One hour and five minutes

Yields: Fourteen servings

Nutrition Facts: Calories: 550.2 | Protein: 8.3g | Carbs: 51.2g| Fat: 32.3g | Fiber: 2.1g

Ingredients

- One and a half cup of chocolate chip cookies
- One-fourth cup of sugar
- One-third cup of butter (melted)

For the filling:

- One cup of sugar
- Half cup of sour cream
- Three packages of cream cheese (softened)
- Half tsp. of vanilla extract
- Three eggs

For the cookie dough:

- One-fourth cup of each

    o   Sugar

    o   Butter (softened)

    o   Brown sugar

- One tbsp. of water

- One tsp. of vanilla extract

- Half cup of flour

- Two cups of mini choco chips

Method:

1. Combine sugar and cookie crumbs in a bowl; add butter. Press the mixture on the bottom of a pan.

2. Combine sugar along with cream cheese in a bowl. Add vanilla and sour cream. Add the eggs and mix well. Pour the mixture over the crust.

3. Cream sugar and butter in another bowl. Add vanilla and water. Add flour along with chocolate chips.

4. Pour the chocolate chip mixture over the layer of cream cheese.

5. Smoothen the surface and bake for fifty minutes.

6. Run a sharp knife along the edges for removing the cake.

Turtle Cheesecake (The Cheesecake Factory)

Total Prep & Cooking Time: Twenty-five minutes

Yields: Eight servings

Nutrition Facts: Calories: 578.3 | Protein: 7.2g | Carbs: 51.3g| Fat: 38.6g | Fiber: 1.2g

Ingredients

- One New York-style cheesecake (frozen, thawed)
- Half cup of each
  - Whipping cream
  - Semisweet chocolate chips
  - Brown sugar
- Three tbsps. of chopped pecans
- One-fourth cup of butter (cubed)
- One tbsp. of light corn syrup

Method:

1. Place the cake on a plate.
2. Melt chocolate chips with one-fourth cup of cream in a bowl; pour it over the cake. Sprinkle pecans from the top.

3. Mix brown sugar, butter, and corn syrup in a pan. Add the remaining cream. Drizzle over the cake.

Tiramisu (Olive Garden)

Total Prep & Cooking Time: One hour and thirty minutes

Yields: Twelve servings

Nutrition Facts: Calories: 172.3 | Protein: 5.4g | Carbs: 18.3g| Fat: 7.2g | Fiber: 0.4g

Ingredients

- Three cups of strong coffee

- Two large eggs (whites and yolks separated)

- One-fourth cup of sugar

- Eight ounces of mascarpone cheese

- One cup of whipping cream

- Three tbsps. of coffee liqueur

- Seven ounces of ladyfingers

- Cocoa powder (to dust)

Method:

1. Combine sugar along with egg yolks in a large bowl. Mix until the mixture becomes thick and pale.

2. Add mascarpone cheese and mix well.

3. Mix egg whites and cream in another bowl for eight minutes. Fold this mixture gently into the mixture of cheese.

4. Combine coffee and liqueur in a bowl.

5. Soak the ladyfingers in the coffee. Arrange half of them as the base of a baking dish. Top with the cheese mixture. Add another layer of ladyfingers. Top with the remaining cheese mixture and smoothen the surface.

6. Dust with the cocoa powder. Refrigerate for one hour or overnight.

Peanut Butter Pie (Bob Evans)

Total Prep & Cooking Time: Three hours and thirty minutes

Yields: Eight servings

Nutrition Facts: Calories: 172.3 | Protein: 5.4g | Carbs: 9.8g| Fat: 12.3g | Fiber: 2.6g

Ingredients

- Five ounces of instant vanilla pudding
- Two cups of whole milk
- Half cup of whipping cream
- Two cups of peanut butter
- One pie shell (baked)
- One jar of hot fudge
- Eight ounces of Cool Whip

Method:

1. Combine pudding mix along with milk in a large bowl. Add cream and peanut butter. Mix well.

2. Add hot fudge onto the bottom of a pie shell. Top with the mixture of pudding.

3. Add Cool Whip as the topping.

4. Refrigerate for one hour.

Triple Fudge Brownie (McAlister's Deli)

Total Prep & Cooking Time: Forty minutes

Yields: Eight servings

Nutrition Facts: Calories: 93.6 | Protein: 1.6g | Carbs: 14.2g| Fat: 3.6g | Fiber: 1.5g

Ingredients

- One package of instant chocolate pudding mix

- One package of chocolate cake mix

- Two cups of semisweet chocolate chips

- Confectioners' sugar

- Vanilla ice cream (to serve)

Method:

1. Start by making the chocolate pudding by following the instructions on the package.

2. Add the chocolate cake mix; add the semisweet chocolate chips. Mix well for combining.

3. Grease a baking dish with cooking spray. Pour the mixture of brownie into the prepared baking dish.

4. Bake for thirty minutes at one-hundred and seventy-five degrees Celsius.

5. Let the brownie sit for ten minutes.

6. Dust using confectioners' sugar.

7. Cut the brownie in squares. Serve with vanilla ice cream.

Note: You can use chopped chocolate chunks for extra flavor and texture.

Coca Cola Cake (Cracker Barrel)

Total Prep & Cooking Time: One hour and five minutes

Yields: Twelve servings

Nutrition Facts: Calories: 608.3 | Protein: 4.3g | Carbs: 91.3g| Fat: 24.6g | Fiber: 1.7g

Ingredients

- One cup of coca-cola
- Half cup of each
    - Unsalted butter
    - Vegetable oil
- Three tbsps. of cocoa powder
- Two cups of each
    - Flour
    - Sugar
- Half tsp. of salt
- One tsp. of baking soda
- Two large eggs
- Half cup of buttermilk
- Two tsps. of vanilla extract

146

For the frosting:

- Half cup of butter

- Two tbsps. of cocoa powder

- Six tbsps. of milk

- One tsp. of vanilla extract

- Four cups of powdered sugar

Method:

1. Preheat your oven at one-hundred and seventy degrees Celsius.

2. Grease a baking dish with cooking spray.

3. Combine flour, baking soda, sugar, and salt in a bowl.

4. Combine oil, cocoa cola, cocoa powder, and butter in a pan. Pour over the mixture of flour.

5. Add buttermilk, eggs, and vanilla. Beat with a hand blender.

6. Pour the mixture in the baking dish. Bake for thirty minutes.

7. Poke holes on the upper surface of the cake.

8. Combine the frosting ingredients in a saucepan.

9. Pour it over the cake.

10. Let the cake sit for thirty minutes.

Strawberry Banana Smoothie (McDonald's)

Total Prep & Cooking Time: Twenty minutes

Yields: Two servings

Nutrition Facts: Calories: 204.5 | Protein: 4.3g | Carbs: 41.3 g| Fat: 3.3g | Fiber: 5.3g

Ingredients

- Half cup of strawberries (frozen)

- One cup of banana (cubed)

- One-third cup of skimmed milk

- Two tsps. of vanilla extract

- One tbsp. of caster sugar

Method:

1. Combine all the listed ingredients in a high power blender.

2. Serve immediately.

Green Apple Sangria (Olive Garden)

Total Prep & Cooking Time: Fifteen minutes

Yields: Six servings

Nutrition Facts: Calories: 208.3 | Protein: 0.3g | Carbs: 32.6g| Fat: 1.3g | Fiber: 0.7g

Ingredients

- Two cups of Moscato
- Six ounces of pineapple juice
- Five ounces of apple puree
- Eight cups of ice
- Half cup of each
    - Orange slices
    - Strawberries
    - Green apple slices

Method:

1. Combine all the ingredients in a pitcher.
2. Serve in glasses with ice cubes.

PART 2:
COPYCAT RECIPES
FROM MEXICO

Mexican cuisine is known for its simplicity, along with the wonderful taste that can take you to a ride of flavorful paradise. Burrito is a common dish of Mexico that can be found in almost all Mexican restaurants. In this chapter, I have included various types of Mexican dishes from all over Mexico that can be made easily.

CHAPTER 1: BREAKFAST RECIPES

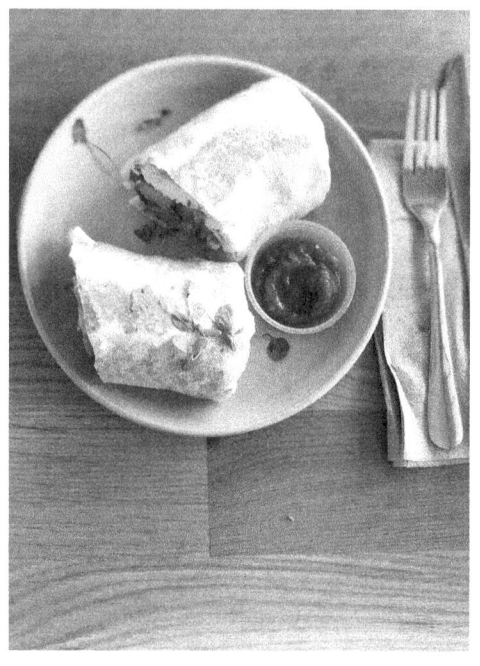

Baked Chimichangas (El Cardenal Alameda)

Total Prep & Cooking Time: Thirty minutes

Yields: Six servings

Nutrition Facts: Calories: 412.3 | Protein: 28.6g | Carbs: 47.2g| Fat: 10.3g | Fiber: 3.3g

Ingredients

- Two cups of chicken breast (cooked, shredded)

- One cup of salsa

- One onion (chopped)

- Three-fourth tsp. of cumin (ground)

- Half tsp. of oregano (dried)

- Six tortillas (warmed)

- Three-fourth cup of cheddar cheese (shredded)

- One cup of chicken stock

- Two tsps. of chicken bouillon granules

- One-eighth tsp. of black pepper

- One-fourth cup of flour

- One-third cup of half and half

- One can of green chilies (chopped)

Method:

1. Preheat your oven at two-hundred degrees Celsius.

2. Take a skillet and add salsa, chicken, cumin, onion, and oregano. Cook until the liquid evaporates.

3. Add half cup of the chicken mixture in the center of each tortilla. Top the chicken with two tbsps. of cheese. Fold the sides and roll the tortillas.

4. Arrange the rolled tortillas in a large baking dish. Bake for fifteen minutes.

5. Mix pepper, bouillon granules, and chicken stock in a pan.

6. Mix cream and flour in a bowl.

7. Add the flour mixture in the pan. Stir well and cook for two minutes.

8. Add the chilies.

9. Serve the chimichangas with sauce from the top.

Spinach Burritos (Café Nin)

Total Prep & Cooking Time: Forty-five minutes

Yields: Six servings

Nutrition Facts: Calories: 380.1 | Protein: 17.9g | Carbs: 40.2g| Fat: 14.5g | Fiber: 4.1g

Ingredients

- Half cup of onion (chopped)
- Two cloves of garlic (minced)
- Two tsps. of butter
- Ten ounces of spinach (chopped, squeezed)
- One-eighth tsp. of pepper
- Six tortillas (warmed)
- Three-fourth cup of Picante sauce
- Two cups of cheddar cheese (shredded)

Method:

1. Heat the butter in an iron skillet; add garlic and onion. Sauté for two minutes. Add pepper and spinach. Cook the mixture for three minutes.

2. Add two tbsps. of the onion and spinach mixture in the middle of each tortilla. Top with two tbsps. of cheese and one tbsp. of Picante sauce. Fold the sides and roll the tortilla.

3. Arrange the tortillas in a baking dish with the seam side down. Top the tortilla rolls with cheese and Picante sauce.

4. Bake for twenty minutes.

5. Serve hot.

Breakfast Tacos (Belmondo)

Total Prep & Cooking Time: Thirty minutes

Yields: Three servings

Nutrition Facts: Calories: 422.2 | Protein: 20.3g | Carbs: 37.9g| Fat: 20.3g | Fiber: 1.6g

Ingredients

- One-fourth cup of onion (chopped)

- One jalapeno pepper (chopped)

- One tbsp. of canola oil

- Two corn tortillas (cut in strips)

- Four eggs

- One-fourth tsp. of salt

- One-eighth tsp. of pepper

- Half cup of Monterey jack cheese (shredded)

- One-fourth cup of tomato (chopped)

- Six flour tortillas (warmed)

Method:

1. Heat the oil in a large skillet. Add jalapeno and onion. Cook for three minutes.

2. Add the strips of tortilla. Cook for two minutes.

3. Combine eggs, pepper, and salt in a bowl; add the egg mixture to the skillet. Add tomato and cheese. Cook for three minutes.

4. Add two tbsps. of egg mixture in each tortilla.

5. Serve immediately.

Egg and Chorizo Wrap (El Cardenal Alameda)

Total Prep & Cooking Time: Twenty minutes

Yields: Six servings

Nutrition Facts: Calories: 510.9 | Protein: 27.3g | Carbs: 26.8g| Fat: 31.3g | Fiber: 2.2g

Ingredients

- Twelve ounces of chorizo (fresh)

- Six large eggs

- Two tbsps. of milk

- One cup of cheddar cheese (shredded)

- Six tortillas (warmed)

Method:

1. Begin by removing the chorizo from the casings.

2. Cook the chorizo in a heavy skillet for eight minutes. Break them into crumbles.

3. Combine eggs and milk in a bowl.

4. Add the mixture of eggs to the skillet. Cook for three minutes. Add the cheese. Cook for two minutes.

5. Add half cup of the egg mixture in the center of each tortilla.

6. Roll the tortillas and serve hot.

Sunrise Sausage Enchiladas (El Ocho)

Total Prep & Cooking Time: One hour and ten minutes

Yields: Ten servings

Nutrition Facts: Calories: 390.8 | Protein: 15.2g | Carbs: 28.9g| Fat: 24.5g | Fiber: 2.6g

Ingredients

- One pound of pork sausage
- Two tbsps. of canola oil
- Seven cups of hash brown potatoes (frozen, thawed)
- Half tsp. of each
    - Chili powder
    - Salt
- One-fourth tsp. of each
    - Pepper
    - Cayenne pepper
- One can of green chilies (chopped)
- Two cups of cheddar cheese (shredded)
- Ten flour tortillas
- Two cans of green enchilada sauce

For the toppings:

- Red onion (chopped)

- Sweet red pepper (chopped)

- Cilantro (chopped)

Method:

1. Take a heavy skillet and cook the pork sausage; cook for seven minutes and crumble the sausage. Keep aside.

2. In the same skillet, heat the oil. Add the potatoes and cook for ten minutes. Remove the skillet from heat and add chilies, seasonings, half cup of cheese, and cooked sausage.

3. Add half a cup of the potato mixture in each tortilla. Roll the tortillas.

4. Grease a baking dish with some cooking spray. Arrange the tortillas in the dish with the seam side down. Top the tortilla rolls with enchilada sauce. Refrigerate for thirty minutes.

5. Bake the enchiladas covered for thirty minutes and one-hundred and fifty degrees Celsius. Add remaining cheese from the top and bake for fifteen minutes.

6. Serve the enchiladas immediately with toppings.

Egg Burritos (Eno)

Total Prep & Cooking Time: Twenty-five minutes

Yields: Ten servings

Nutrition Facts: Calories: 370.6 | Protein: 18.5g | Carbs: 28.9g| Fat: 18.2g | Fiber: 2.1g

Ingredients

- Twelve strips of bacon (chopped)

- Twelve large eggs

- Half tsp. of salt

- One-fourth tsp. of pepper

- Ten flour tortillas (warmed)

- Two cups of cheddar cheese (shredded)

- Four green onion (sliced)

Method:

1. In an iron skillet, cook the chopped bacon for two minutes. Drain the bacon on paper towels. Reserve two tbsps. of the drippings.

2. Combine eggs, pepper, and salt in a bowl.

3. Heat the skillet and add the egg mixture. Cook the eggs for four minutes.

4. Add one-fourth cup of the cooked egg mixture in the center of each tortilla. Sprinkle bacon, green onion, and cheese from the top.

5. Roll the tortillas into burritos and serve immediately.

Tortilla Sausage Breakfast Bake (Belmondo)

Total Prep & Cooking Time: Fifty minutes

Yields: Six servings

Nutrition Facts: Calories: 260.2 | Protein: 21.7g | Carbs: 13.4g| Fat: 12.4g | Fiber: 2.6g

Ingredients

- Eight ounces of lean turkey sausage

- Half cup green chili and diced tomato mixture (canned)

- Six corn tortillas

- Half cup of Monterey jack cheese (shredded)

- One-fourth cup of pepper jack cheese (shredded)

- Two green onions (chopped)

- Six large eggs

- Three-fourth cup of milk (fat-free)

- Three-fourth tsp. of paprika

- One-fourth tsp. of cumin (ground)

Method:

1. Preheat your oven at one-hundred and fifty degrees Celsius.

2. Cook the sausage in an iron skillet for six minutes. Crumble the sausage and add the tomato mixture.

3. Use a cooking spray for coating a nine-inch deep pie plate; use half of the tortillas for lining the pie plate. Sprinkle cheese, sausage mixture, and green onion over the tortilla base. Repeat for another layer.

4. Combine milk, eggs, cumin, and paprika in a large bowl. Pour the egg mixture over the tortilla layers.

5. Bake for twenty minutes. Let it sit for ten minutes.

6. Cut in wedges and serve.

Rellenos Breakfast Bake (Saks Polanco)

Total Prep & Cooking Time: Forty-five minutes

Yields: Fifteen servings

Nutrition Facts: Calories: 206.3 | Protein: 9.6g | Carbs: 12.3g| Fat: 12.6g | Fiber: 1.5g

Ingredients

- Twenty ounces of hash brown potatoes (frozen, shredded)

- One can of green chilies

- One cup of salsa (chunky)

- One pound of fresh chorizo (cooked, crumbled)

- Two cups of Mexican cheese blend (shredded)

- Six large eggs

- Half cup of milk

- One-fourth tsp. of cumin (ground)

- Pepper and salt (for seasoning)

Method:

1. Preheat your oven at one-hundred and fifty degrees Celsius.

2. Grease a baking dish with cooking spray. Layer half of the potatoes as the base of the baking dish. Open the chilies and layer them over the potatoes. Add half of the sausage and half of the cheese.

3. Cover the cheese layer with remaining sausage, potatoes, and cheese.

4. Beat milk and eggs in a bowl; add pepper, cumin, and salt. Pour the mixture over the mixture of potatoes.

5. Bake for forty minutes until the eggs are set properly.

6. Let the dish sit for fifteen minutes.

7. Serve warm.

Mexican Cornbread and Sausage Strata (Delirio)

Total Prep & Cooking Time: One hour and thirty minutes

Yields: Eight servings

Nutrition Facts: Calories: 512.3 | Protein: 17.5g | Carbs: 55.2g| Fat: 34.7g | Fiber: 1.8g

Ingredients

- One pound of chorizo (fresh)

- One onion (chopped)

- One cup of corn (frozen, thawed)

- One and a half cup of pico de gallo (drained)

- Eight cups of cornbread (crumbled coarsely)

- Eight large eggs

- Two cups of milk

- Half tsp. of salt

- One tsp. of garlic powder

- One-eighth tsp. of pepper

- One-third cup of Mexican cheese blend

Method:

1. Heat oil in an iron skillet. Add the chorizo. Cook for seven minutes. Crumble the chorizo using a spatula.

2. Combine the chorizo, pico de gallo, and corn in a bowl. Add the cornbread. Mix well; pour the mixture in a well-greased baking dish.

3. Whisk together salt, eggs, milk, pepper, and garlic powder in another bowl. Pour the egg mixture over the mixture of cornbread.

4. Refrigerate for one hour.

5. Preheat your oven at two hundred degrees Celsius. Bake for forty minutes.

6. Sprinkle cheese from the top.

7. Bake for five minutes.

8. Let the dish sit for ten minutes.

9. Serve warm.

CHAPTER 2:
SNACK AND SIDE DISH RECIPES

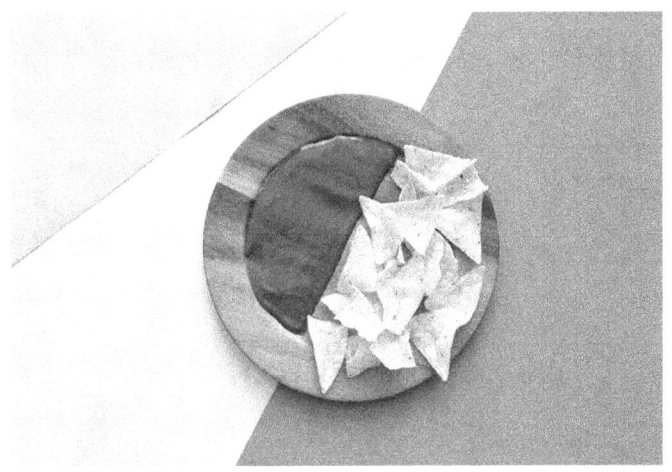

City Ceviche (Pujol)

Total Prep & Cooking Time: One hour and thirty-five minutes

Yields: Twelve servings

Nutrition Facts: Calories: 82.3 | Protein: 7.1g | Carbs: 5.2g| Fat: 4.2g | Fiber: 1.7g

Ingredients

- Half pound of each
    - Sea scallops
    - Shrimp (deveined)
- Half cup of each
    - Lime juice
    - Red onion (sliced)
    - Cilantro (chopped)
- Two tbsps. of orange juice
- One tbsp. of orange zest (grated)
- One red bell pepper (chopped)
- One yellow bell pepper (chopped)
- One cup of tomato (diced)
- One Serrano chili pepper (minced)

- One pinch of salt

- One-eighth tsp. of each

  o Cayenne pepper

  o Cumin (ground)

- One avocado (diced)

- One tbsp. of olive oil

Method:

1. Slice the scallops in half by removing the side muscles.

2. Fill a saucepan with water along with one pinch of salt. Boil the water and add the scallops. Poach the scallops for one minute. Transfer the scallops in ice-cold water.

3. Add shrimps in the same water and cook for two minutes. Transfer the shrimps in ice-cold water.

4. Pat dry the shrimps and scallops. Add them in a bowl along with orange juice and lemon juice. Mix well. Keep in the refrigerator for thirty minutes.

5. Add orange zest, red bell pepper, yellow bell pepper, red onion, chili pepper, tomato, cumin, salt, cilantro, and cayenne in a bowl. Mix well.

6. Add the shrimp and scallop mixture. Stir well.

7. Refrigerate for ten minutes.

8. Add avocado and olive oil. Mix well.

9. Serve in margarita glasses.

Great Chicken Taquitos (Quattro)

Total Prep & Cooking Time: One hour

Yields: Six servings

Nutrition Facts: Calories: 310.3 | Protein: 15.6g | Carbs: 25.1g| Fat: 13.7g | Fiber: 4.6g

Ingredients

- One cup of water
- One pound of chicken breast halves
- Four cups of vegetable oil
- One cup of tomatoes (chopped)
- Half cup of green onion (minced)
- Six tbsps. of chicken stock
- Two tsps. of flour
- One tsp. of garlic (minced)
- Half tsp. of each
    - Cumin (ground)
    - Oregano (dried)
    - Chili powder
    - Salt

- Twelve corn tortillas

- Twelve wooden picks

- One-third cup of lettuce (shredded)

- One-fourth cup of guacamole

Method:

1. Simmer water in a large skillet. Add the breasts of chicken. Cook for twenty minutes. Drain the water and shred the chicken.

2. Take an iron skillet. Heat one tbsp. of oil. Add tomatoes, chicken, chicken stock, green onion, garlic, flour, oregano, chili powder, cumin, and salt. Mix well. Cook for five minutes.

3. Take another skillet and add oil in it. Dip the corn tortillas in the oil for softening them. Drain excess oil using paper towels.

4. Heat oil in a large pan.

5. Add two tbsps. of the chicken mixture in each tortilla. Fold the sides and roll the tortillas. Secure using wooden picks.

6. Fly the rolled tortillas in hot oil for five minutes.

7. Serve the taquitos on lettuce bed and guacamole by the side.

Corn Tortilla Chips (Quintonil)

Total Prep & Cooking Time: Thirty minutes

Yields: Twelve servings

Nutrition Facts: Calories: 123.5 | Protein: 1.4g | Carbs: 13.4g| Fat: 7.2g | Fiber: 1.9g

Ingredients

- Two cups of oil

- Twelve ounces of corn tortillas (cut in six wedges from each)

- Salt (for seasoning)

Method:

1. Heat the oil in a large pan.

2. Add the tortilla wedges. Fry until crisp. Drain excess oil using paper towels.

3. Toss the chips with salt.

4. Serve immediately.

Fried Stuffed Potatoes (Pujol)

Total Prep & Cooking Time: Four hours and fifteen minutes

Yields: Twelve servings

Nutrition Facts: Calories: 360.8 | Protein: 13.4g | Carbs: 44.2g| Fat: 14.5g | Fiber: 3.6g

Ingredients

- Four large potatoes (cubed)

- Half tsp. of salt

- One tbsp. of oil

- Half cup of onion (chopped)

- One green bell pepper (chopped)

- Three garlic cloves (minced)

- One pound of beef (ground)

- Two tsps. of cumin (ground)

- One tsp. of black pepper (ground)

- Four tsps. of tomato pastc

- One-third tbsp. of white vinegar

- Four large eggs

- Two cups of bread crumbs

- One cup of flour

- Two cups of oil (to fry)

Method:

1. Boil the potatoes in salted water for twenty minutes. Drain the water and mash the potatoes in a bowl. Add half tsp. of salt. Mash again.

2. Take a skillet and add onion, garlic, and green pepper. Cook for eight minutes. Add the beef and cook for two minutes. Add pepper, salt, cumin, vinegar, and tomato paste. Mix well. Keep aside.

3. Use waxed paper for lining a baking sheet.

4. Beat the eggs in a bowl. Arrange flour and bread crumbs in separate dishes.

5. Take a handful of mashed potatoes and split them into half; make bowls from each half and fill in the beef mixture. Join the halves and make a round ball. Repeat for the remaining potato and beef.

6. Roll the potato balls in flour and dip in the eggs; roll the balls in bread crumbs. Arrange the balls in the baking sheet. Refrigerate for three hours.

7. Heat oil in a deep pan. Fry the potato balls until crisp.

8. Serve hot.

Chicken Enchilada Nachos (Nana)

Total Prep & Cooking Time: Twenty-five minutes

Yields: Two servings

Nutrition Facts: Calories: 551.3 | Protein: 22.3g | Carbs: 26.8g| Fat: 35.8g | Fiber: 2.7g

Ingredients

- Three tbsps. of butter
- One-fourth cup of onion (chopped)
- One jalapeno pepper (chopped)
- One chili pepper (chopped)
- Two garlic cloves (chopped)
- Half cup of chicken stock
- One chicken breast (cubed)
- One-fourth tsp. of each
    - Chili powder
    - Seasoned salt
    - Cumin (ground)
    - Cayenne pepper
- One tbsp. of flour

- Two tbsps. of sour cream

- One-third cup of pepper jack cheese (shredded)

- Two cups of tortilla chips

- One and a half tbsp. of pico de gallo

Method:

1. Take a skillet. Add two tbsps. of butter. Add jalapeno pepper, onion, chili pepper, and garlic. Fry for three minutes.

2. Add chicken, chicken stock, seasoned salt, chili powder, cayenne pepper, and cumin. Cook for five minutes.

3. Add one tbsp. of butter in a casserole bowl. Microwave for twenty seconds. Add flour and mix until smooth.

4. Add sour cream and flour mixture in the chicken mixture. Cook for four minutes. Add cheese and stir for three minutes.

5. On a large plate, arrange the tortillas chips. Top with pico de gallo and chicken mixture.

Fresco Salsa (Quattro)

Total Prep & Cooking Time: Fifteen minutes

Yields: Twelve servings

Nutrition Facts: Calories: 15.7 | Protein: 0.8g | Carbs: 5.1g| Fat: 0.3g | Fiber: 1.2g

Ingredients

- Six Roma tomatoes (diced)

- One onion (diced)

- One red bell pepper (diced)

- One yellow bell pepper (diced)

- One bunch of cilantro (minced)

- One lime (juiced)

- One tsp. of salt

Method:

1. Mix tomatoes, onion, bell peppers, cilantro, salt, and lime juice in a large bowl.

2. Refrigerate for ten minutes.

3. Serve immediately.

Shrimp Bites (Porfirio's Coapa)

Total Prep & Cooking Time: Ten minutes

Yields: Ten servings

Nutrition Facts: Calories: 60.3 | Protein: 12.3g | Carbs: 2.2g| Fat: 3.6g | Fiber: 1.1g

Ingredients

- Eighteen small shrimps
- Half tsp. of chili powder
- Two tsps. of olive oil
- Three-fourth cup of guacamole
- Eighteen potato chips

Method:

1. Sprinkle chili powder over the shrimps.
2. Heat oil in a skillet. Cook the shrimps for three minutes.
3. Top the chips with guacamole.
4. Top with shrimp.

Spicy Bean Salsa (Meroma)

Total Prep & Cooking Time: Eight hours and ten minutes

Yields: Twelve servings

Nutrition Facts: Calories: 150.3 | Protein: 5.2g | Carbs: 19.6g| Fat: 6.2g | Fiber: 4.6g

Ingredients

- One can of each
  - Black-eyed peas
  - Black beans
  - Whole kernel corn
  - Jalapeno peppers (diced)
  - Tomatoes (diced)
- Half cup of each
  - Onion (chopped)
  - Green bell pepper (chopped)
- One cup of salad dressing
- Half tsp. of garlic salt

Method:

1. Combine all the ingredients in a large bowl.

2. Refrigerate for eight hours.

CHAPTER 3:
APPETIZER RECIPES

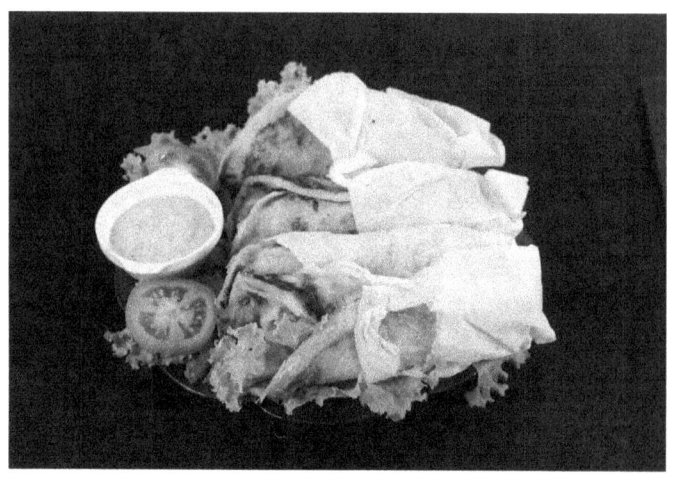

Egg Rolls (Pangea)

Total Prep & Cooking Time: Four hours and thirty minutes

Yields: Five servings

Nutrition Facts: Calories: 418.3 | Protein: 12.5g | Carbs: 20.5g| Fat: 30.1g | Fiber: 2.7g

Ingredients

- Two tbsps. of oil
- One chicken breast
- Two tbsps. of each
    - Green onion (minced)
    - Red bell pepper (minced)
    - Spinach (chopped)
    - Jalapeno peppers (chopped)
- One-third cup of corn kernels (frozen)
- One-fourth cup of black beans (rinsed)
- Two eggs
- Half tbsp. of each
    - Parsley (minced)
    - Cumin (ground)
    - Chili powder

- One-third tsp. of salt

- One pinch of cayenne pepper

- Three-fourth cup of Monterey jack cheese (shredded)

- Five flour tortillas

- Two cups of oil (to fry)

Method:

1. Rub the chicken breast with one tbsp. of oil. Cook the chicken in a pan for five minutes. Dice the chicken.

2. Heat remaining oil in the pan. Add red pepper and onion. Cook for five minutes.

3. Add chicken to the pan along with black beans, corn, eggs, jalapeno peppers, spinach, cumin, parsley, chili powder, cayenne pepper, and salt. Cook for five minutes. Remove the pan from heat; add the cheese. Mix well.

4. Microwave the tortillas for one minute.

5. Spoon the chicken mixture equally in the tortillas; roll the tortillas. Use toothpicks for securing the tortillas. Keep in the refrigerator for four hours.

6. Fry in hot oil for ten minutes.

7. Serve hot.

Cream Cheese Rollups (Nicos)

Total Prep & Cooking Time: One hour and five minutes

Yields: Eight servings

Nutrition Facts: Calories: 412.3 | Protein: 8.6g | Carbs: 41.3g| Fat: 18.5g | Fiber: 3.4g

Ingredients

- Eight ounces of cream cheese (softened)
- One-third cup of mayonnaise
- Two-third cup of green olives (chopped)
- One can of black olives (chopped)
- Eight flour tortillas
- Half cup of salsa

Method:

1. Combine cream cheese, green olives, mayonnaise, green onions, and black olives in a bowl.

2. Spread the cheese mixture in the tortillas; roll the tortillas. Keep in the refrigerator for one hour.

3. Slice the rolled tortillas in one-inch pieces.

4. Serve immediately with salsa.

Antojitos Minis (Pujol)

Total Prep & Cooking Time: Twenty-five minutes

Yields: Twenty-four servings

Nutrition Facts: Calories: 108.3 | Protein: 4.2g | Carbs: 10.4g| Fat: 5.1g | Fiber: 1.3g

Ingredients

- Four flour tortillas
- Three ounces of each
    - Cheddar cheese (shredded)
    - Monterey jack cheese (shredded)
    - White cheddar cheese (shredded)
- One tomato (diced)
- One cup of red bell pepper (diced)
- One-eighth cup of green onions (chopped)
- One-third cup of black beans (drained)
- Two tbsps. of hot salsa
- One-eighth tsp. of chili powder

Method:

1. Preheat your oven at two-hundred degrees Celsius. Grease twelve muffin cups using cooking spray.

2. Cut the tortillas into six round pieces. Insert the round in the muffin cups.

3. Layer white cheddar cheese, cheddar cheese, Monterey jack cheese, red bell pepper, tomato, black beans, green onions, chili powder, and hot salsa in the muffin cups.

4. Bake for five minutes.

5. Serve hot.

Fried Jalapeno Slices (Zefiro)

Total Prep & Cooking Time: Fifteen minutes

Yields: Eight servings

Nutrition Facts: Calories: 145.6 | Protein: 3.8g | Carbs: 14.5g| Fat: 7.1g | Fiber: 1.6g

Ingredients

- One cup of flour
- One tsp. of each
    - Salt
    - Black pepper (ground)
    - Chili powder
    - Garlic powder
- Two large eggs
- One cup of beer
- One and a half cup of oil
- Two cups of jalapeno peppers (sliced)

Method:

1. Combine salt, flour, pepper, garlic powder, red chili powder, beer, and eggs in a bowl.

2. Heat oil in a large pot.

3. Dip the slices of jalapeno in the batter and fry them in the hot oil. Fry until crispy.

4. Serve hot.

Super Nachos (Quintonil)

Total Prep & Cooking Time: Fifty minutes

Yields: Twelve servings

Nutrition Facts: Calories: 430.1 | Protein: 14.3g | Carbs: 38.6g| Fat: 22.6g | Fiber: 5.7g

Ingredients

- One pound of beef (ground)

- Two ounces of taco seasoning mix

- Three-fourth cup of water

- Eighteen ounces of tortilla chips

- One cup of cheddar cheese (shredded)

- One can of refried beans

- Half cup of salsa

- One-third cup of sour cream

- Half a can of black olives (chopped)

- Four green onions (diced)

- Four ounces of jalapeno peppers (sliced)

Method:

1. Cook the beef in an iron skillet for ten minutes. Crumble the beef.

2. Add water and taco seasoning mix. Simmer for ten minutes.

3. Preheat your oven broiler. Use aluminum foil for lining a baking sheet.

4. Arrange the tortilla chips on the baking sheet. Top with cheese, beef mixture, and refried beans.

5. Broil for five minutes.

6. Top with sour cream, salsa, jalapeno peppers, olives, and green onions.

Shrimp Salsa (Nicos)

Total Prep & Cooking Time: One hour and twenty minutes

Yields: Twelve servings

Nutrition Facts: Calories: 27.2 | Protein: 4.3g | Carbs: 1.6g| Fat: 0.5g | Fiber: 0.4g

Ingredients

- Half pound of salad shrimp
- Two tomatoes (diced)
- Half red onion (diced)
- One-fourth cup of cilantro (minced)
- One-third cup of lime juice
- One tsp. of each
    - Black pepper (ground)
    - Salt
- One garlic clove (minced)

Method:

1. Combine shrimp, onion, tomatoes, cilantro, pepper, salt, and lime juice in a bowl.
2. Refrigerate for one hour.
3. Serve cold with extra lemon juice.

Armadillo Eggs (Pangea)

Total Prep & Cooking Time: Fifty-five minutes

Yields: Twelve servings

Nutrition Facts: Calories: 539.6 | Protein: 21.4g | Carbs: 14.6g| Fat: 41.9g | Fiber: 1.4g

Ingredients

- Twenty-four jalapeno peppers

- One pound of sausage

- Two cups of baking mix

- Sixteen ounces of cheddar cheese (shredded)

- One tbsp. of red pepper flakes

- One and a half tbsp. of garlic salt

- Fourteen ounces of Monterey jack cheese (cubed)

Method:

1. Preheat your oven at one-hundred and fifty degrees Celsius. Use a cooking spray for lightly greasing a baking tray.

2. Cut a slit in the peppers. Remove the pulp and seeds.

3. Combine baking mix, sausage, pepper flakes, cheddar cheese, and garlic salt in a bowl.

4. Stuff the cubes of Monterey jack cheese into the jalapeno peppers. Take a handful of the sausage mixture and shape it around the peppers for forming balls.

5. Bake the peppers for twenty minutes.

6. Serve immediately.

Mexican Meatballs (La Distral)

Total Prep & Cooking Time: One hour and ten minutes

Yields: Twenty servings

Nutrition Facts: Calories: 240.3 | Protein: 14.3g | Carbs: 9.6g| Fat: 14.8g | Fiber: 1.4g

Ingredients

- Two pounds of each

    o Beef (ground)

    o Pork (ground)

- Two large eggs

- One and a half cup of bread crumbs

- One tsp. of each

    o Black pepper (ground)

    o Salt

- Two garlic cloves (minced)

- Half cup of water

- Two cans of diced tomato

- Three chipotle peppers in adobo sauce

- Four tsps. of oil

- Two onions (diced)

- Two tsps. of cumin (ground)

- Two cups of chicken stock

- One cup of cilantro (chopped)

Method:

1. Combine pork, beef, bread crumbs, eggs, pepper, salt, minced garlic, and water in a bowl. Mix well and form meatballs of one-inch.

2. Blend diced tomatoes with chipotle peppers in a food processor.

3. Heat oil in a large pan. Add the onions. Cook for two minutes. Add cumin and remaining garlic; add tomato mixture along with the chicken stock. Simmer for five minutes.

4. Heat oil in another skillet. Add the meatballs and fry until browned.

5. Add the meatballs in the sauce and simmer for thirty seconds.

6. Garnish with cilantro and serve.

Chicken Wonton Tacos (El Cardenal Alameda)

Total Prep & Cooking Time: One hour and thirty minutes

Yields: Six servings

Nutrition Facts: Calories: 240.6 | Protein: 15.7g | Carbs: 20.1g| Fat: 9.6g | Fiber: 2.6g

Ingredients

- One head of red cabbage (chopped)

- Four carrots (grated)

- One-fourth cup of each

    o Red wine vinegar

    o Coleslaw dressing

    o Stir-fry sauce

- Two tbsps. of each

    o Teriyaki sauce

    o Soy sauce

    o Sesame oil

- One pound of chicken (ground)

- Twelve wonton wrappers

Method:

1. Combine carrots, cabbage, vinegar, coleslaw dressing, soy sauce, and teriyaki sauce in a bowl. Refrigerate for one hour.

2. Preheat your oven at one-hundred and seventy-five degrees Celsius.

3. Heat the oil in an iron skillet. Cook the chicken for seven minutes. Add the stir-fry sauce. Simmer for two minutes.

4. Shape the wrappers like tacos by placing them between muffin cups. Bake for five minutes.

5. Add two tbsps. of the chicken mixture and top with the slaw.

6. Serve immediately.

Monkey Bread (Meroma)

Total Prep & Cooking Time: Fifty-five minutes

Yields: Twelve servings

Nutrition Facts: Calories: 190.4 | Protein: 6.3g | Carbs: 16.7g| Fat: 11.2g | Fiber: 0.6g

Ingredients

- Two tbsps. of butter (melted)

- Sixteen ounces of buttermilk biscuit dough (separated, cut in quarters)

- One and a half cup of cheddar cheese (shredded)

- Three-fourth cup of jalapeno pepper (sliced)

- Three-fourth tsp. of parsley flakes

- One cup of mozzarella cheese (shredded)

Method:

1. Preheat your oven at one-hundred and fifty degrees Celsius. Grease a loaf pan using cooking spray.

2. Dip the pieces of the dough in the melted butter.

3. Layer the dough pieces as a base in the load pan. Top with one-fourth cup of pepper, half cup of cheese, and one-fourth tsp. of parsley. Repeat for the remaining layers.

4. Mix the leftover cheddar cheese with mozzarella cheese. Spread the mixture over the ingredients.

5. Bake for forty minutes.

CHAPTER 4:
SOUP RECIPES

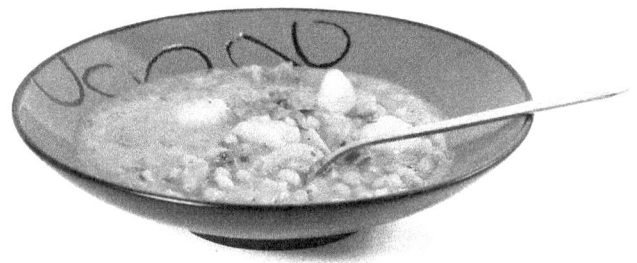

Taco Soup (Testal)

Total Prep & Cooking Time: Twenty-five minutes

Yields: Eight servings

Nutrition Facts: Calories: 367.9 | Protein: 26.3g | Carbs: 34.3g| Fat: 13.5g | Fiber: 7.2g

Ingredients

- Two pounds of beef (ground)

- One pack of taco seasoning

- Two cups of water

- One can of mild chili beans

- Fifteen ounces of whole kernel corn (drained)

- Fourteen ounces of pinto beans (rinsed)

- Twelve ounces of stewed potatoes

- Ten ounces of diced tomato and chili

- Four ounces of green chilies (chopped)

- One envelope of ranch dressing mix

Method:

1. Cook the beef in a large pot for ten minutes.

2. Add the remaining ingredients. Boil and simmer for fifteen minutes.

3. Serve hot.

Corn Chicken Chowder (La Vicenta Vallejo)

Total Prep & Cooking Time: Thirty minutes

Yields: Eight servings

Nutrition Facts: Calories: 360.3 | Protein: 22.8g | Carbs: 13.2g| Fat: 22.6g | Fiber: 1.9g

Ingredients

- Two pounds of chicken breast (cut in pieces of one-inch)

- Half cup of onion (chopped)

- Three tbsps. of butter

- Two cloves of garlic (minced)

- One cup of hot water

- Two tsps. of chicken bouillon granules

- One tsp. of cumin (ground)

- Two cups of half and half

- One and a half cup of Monterey jack cheese (shredded)

- One can of cream-style corn

- Four ounces of green chilies (chopped)

- One-fourth tsp. of hot pepper sauce

- One tomato (chopped)

Method:

1. Cook the onion and chicken in a large pan along with butter. Add the garlic, cumin, bouillon granules, and water. Simmer for five minutes.

2. Add cheese, cream, chilies, corn, and hot sauce. Add the tomato and simmer for two minutes.

3. Garnish with cilantro.

Cream White Chili (Porfirio's Coapa)

Total Prep & Cooking Time: Fifty minutes

Yields: Seven servings

Nutrition Facts: Calories: 331.3 | Protein: 21.2g | Carbs: 23.6g| Fat: 15.6g | Fiber: 7.2g

Ingredients

- One pound of chicken breast (cut in cubes of half-inch)

- One onion (chopped)

- Two tsps. of garlic powder

- One tbsp. of canola oil

- Two cans of beans (rinsed)

- One can of chicken stock

- Two and a half can of green chilies (chopped)

- One tsp. of each

    o Oregano (dried)

    o Salt

    o Cumin (ground

    o Pepper

- One-fourth tsp. of cayenne pepper

- One cup of sour cream

- Half cup of whipping cream

Method:

1. Sauté onion, chicken, and garlic powder in a large saucepan; add chicken stock, beans, seasonings, and chilies. Boil and simmer for thirty minutes.

2. Add whipping cream and sour cream.

3. Serve hot.

Refried Bean Soup (Pujol)

Total Prep & Cooking Time: Thirty minutes

Yields: Eight servings

Nutrition Facts: Calories: 115.7 | Protein: 4.5g | Carbs: 22.1g| Fat: 1.6g | Fiber: 4.8g

Ingredients

- Sixteen ounces of refried beans
- One can of each
    - Whole kernel corn
    - Black beans
    - Chicken stock
    - Stewed tomatoes
- Half cup of water
- Four ounces of green chilies (chopped)
- One-fourth cup of salsa
- Tortilla chips (to serve)

Method:

1. Combine all the ingredients except for the tortilla chips in a saucepan. Simmer for ten minutes.
2. Serve the soup with tortilla chips.

Chicken Enchilada Soup (Pujol)

Total Prep & Cooking Time: Six hours and thirty minutes

Yields: Eight servings

Nutrition Facts: Calories: 122.5 | Protein: 14.3g | Carbs: 38.6g| Fat: 9.3g | Fiber: 3.3g

Ingredients

- One tbsp. of canola oil

- Two poblano peppers (chopped)

- One onion (chopped)

- Three cloves of garlic (minced)

- One pound of chicken breast

- Forty-eight ounces of chicken stock

- One can of diced tomatoes

- Ten ounces of enchilada sauce

- Two tbsps. of tomato paste

- One tbsp. of chili powder

- Two tsps. of cumin (ground)

- Half tsp. of pepper

- One tsp. of hot pepper sauce

- One-third cup of cilantro (minced)

Method:

1. Heat oil in an iron skillet. Cook onions and pepper for eight minutes. Add minced garlic.

2. Add the chicken and pepper mixture to a slow cooker. Add tomatoes, stock, tomato paste, enchilada sauce, seasonings, and hot sauce. Cook for six hours.

3. Remove the chicken and shred using a fork. Return the shredded chicken to the cooker. Cook for two minutes. Add cilantro.

Big Red Soup (Nana)

Total Prep & Cooking Time: Eight hours and twenty minutes

Yields: Twelve servings

Nutrition Facts: Calories: 112.3 | Protein: 2.3g | Carbs: 22.6g| Fat: 5.6g | Fiber: 1.2g

Ingredients

- Two pounds of beef stew meat (cut in cubes of one-inch)
- Two tbsps. of canola oil
- Three-fourth cup of onion (chopped)
- Two garlic cloves (minced)
- Two cans of diced tomatoes
- One can of beef stock
- Ten ounces of chicken stock
- Twelve ounces of tomato soup
- One-fourth cup of water
- One tsp. of each
  - Cumin (ground)
  - Chili powder

- o Salt

- o Lemon-pepper seasoning

- Two tsps. of Worcestershire sauce

- One-third cup of Picante sauce

- Eight corn tortillas (cut in quarters)

- One cup of cheddar cheese (shredded)

Method:

1. Brown the beef in a saucepan with some oil.

2. Transfer the beef to a slow cooker. Add the remaining listed ingredients except for the cheese and tortillas. Cook for eight minutes.

3. Add tortillas at the bottom of serving bowls. Pour the soup in bowls and top with cheese.

Corn and Chorizo Soup (La Distral)

Total Prep & Cooking Time: Fifty minutes

Yields: Ten servings

Nutrition Facts: Calories: 265.6 | Protein: 12.3g | Carbs: 24.6g| Fat: 14.6g | Fiber: 2.2g

Ingredients

- One pound of chorizo

- One onion (chopped)

- One sweet red pepper (chopped)

- One poblano pepper (chopped)

- Three cloves of garlic (minced)

- One-third cup of flour

- One tsp. of cumin (ground)

- Half tsp. of salt

- One and a half tsp. of pepper

- Two cartons of chicken stock

- Two pounds of potatoes (cut in cubes of half-inch)

- Three cups of corn (frozen)

- Half cup of sour cream

Method:

- Crumble the chorizo in a large skillet. Cook for six minutes. Keep aside.

- Add onion, red peppers, and poblano peppers in the same skillet. Cook for ten minutes. Add garlic, seasonings, and flour. Cook for three minutes. Add the stock.

- Add corn and potatoes; simmer for fifteen minutes. Add chorizo and sour cream.

- Serve hot.

Beefy Rice Soup (Zefiro)

Total Prep & Cooking Time: One hour

Yields: Ten servings

Nutrition Facts: Calories: 390.3 | Protein: 23.5g | Carbs: 29.6g| Fat: 17.9g | Fiber: 6.1g

Ingredients

- Two pounds of beef (ground)

- One-third cup of onion (chopped)

- One tsp. of garlic (minced)

- Three tbsps. of taco seasoning

- Two cups of beef broth

- Two and a half cup of corn (frozen)

- Fifteen ounces of black beans

- Fourteen ounces of diced tomatoes

- One cup of tomato puree

- Two tsps. of each

  - Lime juice

  - Salt

- Half tsp. of cilantro

- One and a half cup of whole grain rice

Method:

1. Cook beef with garlic and onion in a skillet. Add taco seasoning. Add broth, black beans, corn, tomato puree, diced tomatoes, salt, lime juice, rice, and cilantro.

2. Boil and simmer for thirty minutes.

CHAPTER 5:
CHICKEN, PORK, AND
BEEF RECIPES

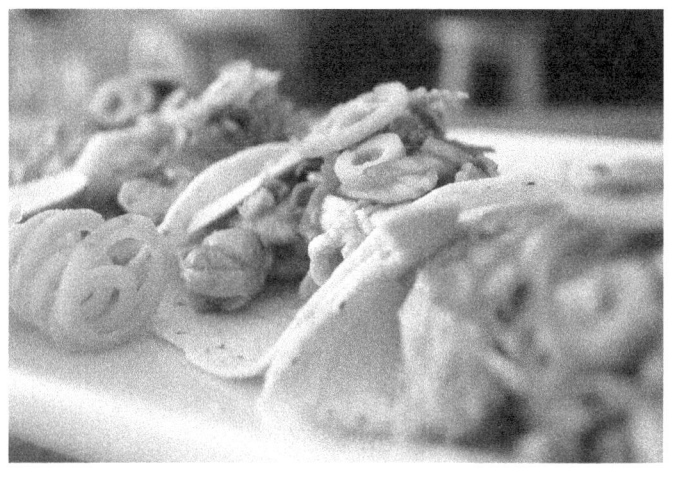

Chicken Tamales (Quintonil)

Total Prep & Cooking Time: Two hours and fifty minutes

Yields: Ten servings

Nutrition Facts: Calories: 246.3 | Protein: 10.3g | Carbs: 21.6g| Fat: 17.6g | Fiber: 5.6g

Ingredients

- Twenty-four corn husks

- One broiler chicken (cut up)

- One onion (quartered)

- Two tsps. of salt

- One clove of garlic (crushed)

- Three cups of water

For the dough:

- One cup of shortening

- Three cups of masa harina

For the filling:

- Six tbsps. of canola oil

- Five tbsps. of flour

- Three-fourth cup of chili powder

- Half tsp. of salt

- One-fourth tsp. of each

  o Pepper

  o Garlic powder

- Two cans of ripe olives (sliced)

Method:

1. Soak the corn husks in cold water. Soak for two hours.

2. Add onion, chicken, garlic, and salt in a pot; add three cups of water. Simmer the mixture for sixty minutes. Remove the chicken and shred. Reserve about six cups of the stock.

3. Beat the shortening for one minute; add the stock and masa harina. Mix well.

4. Heat oil in an iron skillet. Add flour and stir until blended; add remaining stock, chicken, and seasonings. Simmer for forty minutes.

5. Dry the corn husks. Tear four corn husks for making twenty strips for tying.

6. On the husks' wide ends, add tbsps. of the dough and top with two tbsps. of the

chicken mixture. Add two tsps. of olives. Overlap the sides and tie the tamales.

7. Steam the tamales in a steamer for forty-five minutes.

Chicken Mole (Pangea)

Total Prep & Cooking Time: Six hours and twenty minutes

Yields: Twelve servings

Nutrition Facts: Calories: 308.3 | Protein: 25.6g | Carbs: 13.6g| Fat: 17.6g | Fiber: 3.3g

Ingredients

- Twelve chicken thighs
- One tsp. of salt

For the sauce:

- One can of whole tomatoes
- One onion (chopped)
- Two dried chilies
- Half cup of almonds (sliced)
- One-fourth cup of raisin
- Three ounces of bittersweet chocolate (chopped)
- Three tbsps. of olive oil
- One chipotle pepper in adobo sauce
- Three cloves of garlic (halved)

- Three-fourth tsp. of cumin (ground)

- Half tsp. of cinnamon (ground)

Method:

1. Sprinkle the chicken thighs with some salt. Add in a slow cooker.

2. Add onion, tomatoes, almonds, chilies, chocolate, raisins, chipotle pepper, oil, cumin, garlic, and cinnamon in a blender. Blend until smooth. Pour the mixture over the chicken.

3. Cook for six hours.

Chicken Lime Tacos (Meroma)

Total Prep & Cooking Time: Five hours and ten minutes

Yields: Six servings

Nutrition Facts: Calories: 289.6 | Protein: 27.6g | Carbs: 35.8g| Fat: 4.3g | Fiber: 2.6g

Ingredients

- Two pounds of chicken breast halves
- Three tbsps. of lime juice
- One tbsp. of chili powder
- One cup of corn (frozen)
- One cup of chunky salsa
- Twelve flour tortillas (warmed)

Method:

1. Add the chicken in a slow cooker. Mix chili powder along with lime juice in a bowl. Pour the lime mixture over the chicken. Cook for five hours.

2. Shred the chicken and return to the cooker. Add salsa and corn. Cook for thirty minutes.

3. Add the chicken filling in the tortillas and serve.

Chicken Skillet Rice (Pujol)

Total Prep & Cooking Time: Thirty minutes

Yields: Six servings

Nutrition Facts: Calories: 300.2 | Protein: 24.6g | Carbs: 38.6g| Fat: 4.2g | Fiber: 5.2g

Ingredients

- One large egg (beaten)
- One pound of chicken tenderloins (chopped)
- One onion (chopped)
- One tbsp. of olive oil
- Two cloves of garlic (minced)
- Two cups of jasmine rice (cooked)
- One can of black beans (rinsed)
- Eleven ounces of Mexicorn (drained)
- Seven ounces of sweet red peppers (sliced)
- Eight ounces of taco sauce
- Two green onions (chopped)
- One-fourth cup of cilantro (minced)

Method:

1. Cook the egg in a skillet along with some cooking spray. Keep aside.

2. Add onion and chicken in the same skillet. Add the garlic. Cook for one minute.

3. Add beans, rice, Mexicorn, taco sauce, peppers, and green onions. Add the egg.

4. Stir-fry for one minute.

5. Garnish with cilantro.

Pork Burritos (Sonora Grill Amores)

Total Prep & Cooking Time: Three hours

Yields: Twenty servings

Nutrition Facts: Calories: 456.3 | Protein: 17.6g | Carbs: 40.3g| Fat: 21.3g | Fiber: 3.8g

Ingredients

- Three pounds of pork shoulder roast

- One onion (sliced)

- Six garlic cloves (chopped)

- Two ounces of taco seasoning mix

- Six cups of water

- One can of diced tomatoes

- One can of refried beans

- Four ounces of green chilies (chopped)

- Half ounce of taco seasoning mix

- Sixteen ounces of cheddar cheese (shredded)

- Twenty flour tortillas

- One-fourth cup of vegetable oil

Method:

1. Add pork, onion, taco seasoning mix, and garlic in a pot. Cover with water. Simmer for two hours.

2. Shred the pork using a fork. Add refried beans, tomatoes, taco seasoning mix, and green chilies.

3. Add the pork mixture evenly in the tortillas. Top with cheddar cheese. Roll the tortillas for shaping like a burrito.

4. Heat some oil in an iron skillet. Add the burritos and fry for two minutes.

Mexican Slow Cooker Pork (Thiara)

Total Prep & Cooking Time: Eight hours and five minutes

Yields: Twelve servings

Nutrition Facts: Calories: 146.3 | Protein: 24.1g | Carbs: 4.3g| Fat: 3.7g | Fiber: 1.3g

Ingredients

- Four pounds of pork tenderloin (cubed)

- Sixteen ounces of hot Picante sauce

- Seven ounces of green chilies (chopped)

- One can of chipotle peppers

- Two limes (juiced)

Method:

1. Add the pork in a slow cooker; add Picante sauce over the pork. Add chipotle peppers, green chilies, and lime juice.

2. Cook for five hours. Remove the pork and shred. Return the pork in the cooker and cook for three hours.

Tomatoed Pork (Testal)

Total Prep & Cooking Time: One hour

Yields: Six servings

Nutrition Facts: Calories: 242.3 | Protein: 15.6g | Carbs: 4.6g| Fat: 17.3g | Fiber: 1.9g

Ingredients

- Two tbsps. of canola oil
- Two pounds of pork shoulder (cut in chunks of one-inch)
- Two tsps. of each
  - Black pepper (ground)
  - Salt
- Two jalapeno pepper
- One-fourth cup of onion (sliced)
- One garlic clove (crushed)
- Six ounces of mushroom
- One can of diced tomatoes
- Half tsp. of cumin (ground)

Method:

1. Season the pork with pepper and salt.

2. Heat oil in an iron skillet. Add the pork along with jalapeno peppers, cover, and simmer for twenty minutes. Remove the peppers and cook the pork for ten minutes. Chop the peppers.

3. Add garlic and onion. Cook for two minutes. Add mushrooms, jalapeno peppers, and tomatoes. Add the cumin

4. Simmer for ten minutes.

Pork Enchiladas (Nicos)

Total Prep & Cooking Time: Fifty minutes

Yields: Six servings

Nutrition Facts: Calories: 490.5 | Protein: 31.3g | Carbs: 30.6g| Fat: 25.6g | Fiber: 2.3g

Ingredients

- Two cups of cooked pork (shredded)

- Ten ounces of enchilada sauce

- Half tsp. of onion powder

- One cup of sour cream

- One can of green chilies (chopped)

- Two cups of Monterey jack cheese (shredded)

- Twelve ounces of condensed tomato soup

- One-fourth tsp. of garlic powder

- One tsp. of cumin (ground)

- Six flour tortillas

Method:

1. Preheat your oven at one-hundred and fifty degrees Celsius.

2. Mix pork, onion powder, enchilada sauce, half cup of sour cream, one cup of cheese, and green chilies in a bowl.

3. Combine tomato soup, remaining sour cream, cumin, and garlic powder in a bowl.

4. Add a layer of tomato soup mixture in a baking dish.

5. Add the pork mixture in the tortillas. Roll the tortillas. Arrange the tortillas with the seam side down in the layer of tomato soup. Pour over the remaining mixture of soup over the tortillas. Top with cheese.

6. Bake for thirty minutes.

Sizzling Fajitas (Pujol)

Total Prep & Cooking Time: Two hours and forty minutes

Yields: Four servings

Nutrition Facts: Calories: 446.3 | Protein: 25.6g | Carbs: 45.6g| Fat: 20.8g | Fiber: 5.3g

Ingredients

- Four garlic cloves (minced)
- One tbsp. of salt
- Three tbsps. of each
    - Olive oil
    - Lime juice
    - Cilantro (minced)
- One tsp. of chili powder
- Half tsp. of each
    - Paprika
    - White sugar
- One-fourth tsp. of cayenne pepper
- Two pounds of beefsteak (cut in strips of one-fourth inch)
- Six wheat tortillas

- One tbsp. of canola oil
- One onion (sliced)
- One red bell pepper (cut in strips)
- One garlic clove (minced)

Method:

1. Grind salt and garlic using a mortar and pestle.

2. Combine garlic paste, olive oil, lime juice, chili powder, cilantro, paprika, sugar, and cayenne pepper in a bowl. Add the beef and marinate for two hours in the refrigerator.

3. Preheat your oven at one-hundred and fifty degrees Celsius.

4. Wrap the wheat tortillas in an aluminum foil and bake for ten minutes.

5. Heat oil in a pan. Add bell pepper and onion. Cook for five minutes. Keep aside.

6. Add beef in the same pan. Cook for six minutes.

7. Add the mixture of onion and pepper; add salt and garlic. Mix well.

8. Divide the beef strips among warm tortillas.

Beef Tacos and Mango Salsa (La Distral)

Total Prep & Cooking Time: One hour and fifty minutes

Yields: Four servings

Nutrition Facts: Calories: 1120.3 | Protein: 48.5g | Carbs: 162.7g| Fat: 31.8g | Fiber: 21.4g

Ingredients

For the rice and black beans:

- Two tbsps. of olive oil

- One onion (chopped)

- One green bell pepper (chopped)

- Two garlic cloves (minced)

- Five cups of water

- Two cans of black beans (rinsed)

- Three cups of brown rice

- One tsp. of cumin (ground)

- Half tsp. of salt

- One-fourth tsp. of smoked paprika

- One pinch of black pepper

- One bay leaf

For the mango salsa:

- Two cups of mango (chopped)
- One cup of red bell pepper (chopped)
- Two-third cup of green onion (chopped)
- One-fourth cup of cilantro (chopped)
- One jalapeno pepper (minced)
- Two tbsps. of lime juice
- One tbsp. of olive oil

For the filling:

- One pound of ground beef
- One tbsp. of chili powder
- Two tsps. of cumin (ground)
- One-fourth tsp. of each
  - Onion powder
  - Garlic powder
  - Oregano (dried)
  - Paprika
- One pack of flour tortillas

Method:

1. Heat oil in a pan. Add bell pepper, onion, and garlic. Cook for two minutes and add black beans, water, rice, salt, cumin, and paprika. Add the bay leaf; cover the pan and simmer for sixty minutes. Discard the bay leaf.

2. Combine the ingredients for the mango salsa.

3. Heat oil in an iron skillet. Cook beef with cumin, chili powder, onion powder, garlic powder, oregano, red pepper flakes, and paprika. Cook for six minutes.

4. Combine beef mixture with mango and beans mixture. Fill the tortillas.

5. Serve hot.

Bean and Beef Tostadas (Thiara)

Total Prep & Cooking Time: Thirty minutes

Yields: Three servings

Nutrition Facts: Calories: 741.3 | Protein: 36.1g | Carbs: 57.3g| Fat: 35.1g | Fiber: 12.6g

Ingredients

For the beef and bean mixture:

- Half tsp. of each
    - o Onion powder
    - o Garlic salt
    - o Garlic powder
    - o Cumin (ground)
- One-fourth tsp. of black pepper (ground)
- Half pound of beef (ground)
- Half cup of sweet onion (chopped)
- One garlic clove (minced)
- Two cups of refried beans

For the tostada shells:

- Six corn tortillas

- Two tbsps. of vegetable oil

For the garnishing:

- One tomato (diced)

- Two cups of lettuce (shredded)

- One and a half cup of cheddar cheese (shredded)

Method:

1. Preheat your oven at two-hundred degrees Celsius.

2. Combine onion powder, salt, garlic powder, black pepper, and cumin.

3. Heat oil in an iron skillet. Cook the beef for seven minutes with the spice mixture, garlic, and onion.

4. Brush the tortillas with oil on both sides. Bake for five minutes.

5. Heat the beans in a pan for five minutes.

6. Divide the cooked beans among the tostadas. Top with beef mixture and garnishing.

Chipotle Barbacoa (Pangea)

Total Prep & Cooking Time: Six hours and thirty minutes

Yields: Six servings

Nutrition Facts: Calories: 240.3 | Protein: 22.3g | Carbs: 7.1g| Fat: 12.4g | Fiber: 1.6g

Ingredients

- Two tbsps. of vegetable oil
- Two pounds of beef chuck roast (cut in six pieces)
- One-third cup of apple cider
- Four chipotle peppers in adobo sauce
- Three tbsps. of lime juice
- Four cloves of garlic (minced)
- Four tsps. of cumin (ground)
- One Serrano pepper (chopped)
- One tbsp. of cayenne pepper
- Two and a half tsp. of oregano (dried)
- One tsp. of each
  - Garlic powder

- o   Black pepper (ground)
- Half tsp. of each
  - o   Cloves (ground)
  - o   Salt
- One cup of chicken stock
- One onion (chopped)
- Three bay leaves

Method:

1. Heat oil in an iron skillet. Add the beef and cook for ten minutes. Transfer to a slow cooker.

2. Mix all the ingredients in a food processor except for bay leaves, onion, and chicken stock. Blend well. Pour the paste over the beef.

3. Add onion, stock, and bay leaves.

4. Cook for six hours.

5. Shred the pieces of beg using a fork.

Burrito Pie (Testal)

Total Prep & Cooking Time: One hour

Yields: Sixteen servings

Nutrition Facts: Calories: 423.6 | Protein: 18.6g | Carbs: 31.2g| Fat: 21.9g | Fiber: 4.6g

Ingredients

- Two pounds of beef (ground)

- One onion (chopped)

- Two tsps. of garlic (minced)

- Two ounces of black olives (sliced)

- One can of green chili peppers (diced)

- Ten ounces of tomatoes (diced)

- One jar of taco sauce

- Two cans of refried beans

- Twelve flour tortillas

- Nine ounces of Colby cheese (shredded)

Method:

1. Preheat your oven at one-hundred and seventy degrees Celsius.

2. Sauté the beef in an iron skillet. Add garlic and onion. Sauté for five minutes. Add beans, olives, chili peppers, tomatoes, and taco sauce. Cook for twenty minutes

3. Add one layer of the mixture of beef in the base of a baking dish. Cover the meat layer with tortillas and cheese. Repeat for the remaining layers. Top with remaining cheese and meat.

4. Bake for thirty minutes.

CHAPTER 6:
BURGER AND
SANDWICH RECIPES

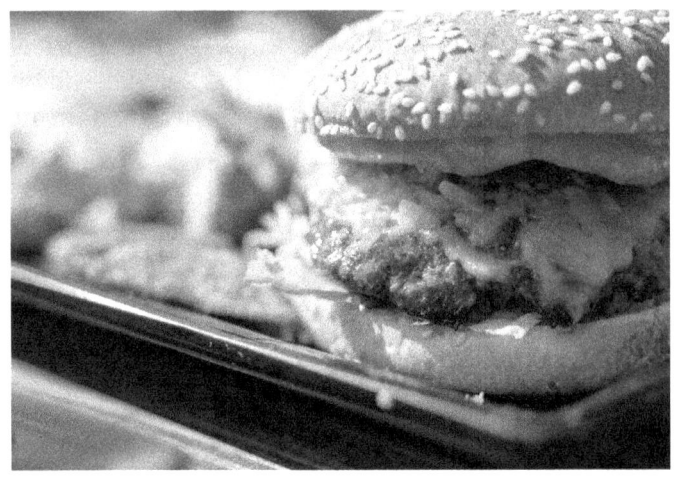

Mexican Grilled Cheese Sandwich (Matcha Mio)

Total Prep & Cooking Time: Twenty-five minutes

Yields: Four servings

Nutrition Facts: Calories: 401.3 | Protein: 10.3g | Carbs: 37.9g| Fat: 21.2g | Fiber: 4.1g

Ingredients

- One sweet yellow pepper (chopped)

- One green pepper (chopped)

- Two tsps. of olive oil

- Eight slices of rye bread

- Two tbsps. of mayonnaise

- One cup of salsa

- Three-fourth cup of Mexican cheese blend

- Two and a half tbsp. of butter (softened)

Method:

1. Sauté the peppers in a small pan in some oil.

2. Spread mayonnaise on four slices of bread. Top with salsa, peppers, and cheese. Add the remaining bread slices on

top. Brush some butter on the outside layer.

3. Toast the sandwiches for five minutes on each side in an iron skillet.

Mexican Grilled Veggie Sandwich (Panaderia Rosetta)

Total Prep & Cooking Time: Thirty minutes

Yields: Four servings

Nutrition Facts: Calories: 359.2 | Protein: 13.5g | Carbs: 54.6g| Fat: 9.6g | Fiber: 6.2g

Ingredients

- One red bell pepper (sliced)

- Two tbsps. of lime juice

- One tbsp. of each

    o Olive oil

    o Oregano

- Half tsp. of each

    o Cumin (ground)

    o Black pepper (ground)

- One-fourth tsp. of each

    o Red pepper (ground)

    o Salt

- One can of black beans

- One zucchini (sliced)

- One red onion (sliced)

- One ciabatta bread loaf (halved)

- Two ounces of pepper jack cheese (shredded)

Method:

1. Preheat your broiler at high settings.

2. Arrange the slices of bell pepper on a baking sheet. Broil for ten minutes.

3. Combine lime juice, oregano, oil, black pepper, beans, and red pepper in a food processor. Blend well.

4. Grease a pan with cooking spray. Grill zucchini and onion slices on the pan for five minutes.

5. Hollow the bottom and top halves of the bread. Arrange a mixture of black beans, onion, zucchini, and bell pepper. Top with salt and cheese. Add the other half of the bread. Use a cooking spray for coating both sides of the bread.

6. Grill on a pan for three minutes on each side.

7. Cut in quarters and serve.

Mexican Torta (Café Nin)

Total Prep & Cooking Time: Thirty minutes

Yields: Four servings

Nutrition Facts: Calories: 560.3 | Protein: 27.5g | Carbs: 52.3g| Fat: 22.6g | Fiber: 3.2g

Ingredients

- Four chicken breast halves

- Four ciabatta rolls

- One-fourth cup of mayonnaise

- One-third cup of refried beans

- Half avocado (mashed)

- Two mozzarella string cheese

- One cup of bread crumbs

- Two large eggs

- Five tbsps. of oil

- One can of pickled jalapenos

Method:

1. Pound the chicken breasts.

2. Heat oil in an iron skillet.

3. Beat the eggs in a bowl. Arrange the bread crumbs in a dish.

4. Dip the pieces of chicken in egg and then coat in bread crumbs.

5. Add the chicken to the pan. Cook for three minutes on each side.

6. Cut the rolls in half. Toast them in a pan.

7. Add mayonnaise on the inside portion of a roll. Layer with refried beans and avocado. Add cooked chicken and top with the other half of the roll.

8. Grill in a pan for three minutes on each side.

Cemita (Pujol)

Total Prep & Cooking Time: Twenty minutes

Yields: One serving

Nutrition Facts: Calories: 870.3 | Protein: 63.2g | Carbs: 71.2g| Fat: 31.7g | Fiber: 8.8g

Ingredients

- One cemita bun

- One tbsp. of adobo sauce

- Two chipotle peppers (cut in strips)

- One-fourth cup of Mexican pulled pork (cooked)

- One and a half tbsp. of cilantro (chopped)

- One-third cup of Mexican string cheese (shredded)

- Four tomato slices

- Half avocado (sliced)

Method:

1. Slice the bun in half.

2. Add half tbsp. of adobo sauce on each side of the bun. Add half of the chipotle peppers on the buns.

3. Add the pulled pork on the bottom bun. Top with cilantro, cheese, avocado, and tomato.

4. Top with another half of the bun.

Mexican-Style Cheeseburger (El Beneficio Cafe)

Total Prep & Cooking Time: Twenty minutes

Yields: Four servings

Nutrition Facts: Calories: 980.1 | Protein: 51.3g | Carbs: 114.3g| Fat: 67.4g | Fiber: 15.6g

Ingredients

- Two pounds of beef (ground)

- One large egg

- One-fourth cup of cornmeal

- Half cup of salsa

- One-third cup of cheddar cheese (grated)

- Three tbsp. green chilies (chopped)

- One cup of cilantro (chopped)

- One tsp. of each

  o Onion powder

  o Garlic powder

- Half tsp. of each

  o Salt

  o Cumin (ground)

        o   Black pepper (ground)

- Four sesame buns

For the toppings:

- Guacamole

- Onion rings

- Slices of cheddar cheese

- Lettuce

Method:

1. Combine all the ingredients in a large bowl. Make four patties from the mixture.

2. Heat oil in an iron skillet and sear the patties for eight minutes on each side.

3. Cut the buns in half. Layer with guacamole, lettuce, beef patty, onion rings, and cheese.

Spicy Burger (Thiara)

Total Prep & Cooking Time: Thirty minutes

Yields: Four servings

Nutrition Facts: Calories: 763.3 | Protein: 41.5g | Carbs: 48.5g| Fat: 36.8g | Fiber: 5.4g

Ingredients

- One dried chili
- Apple cider vinegar (as per requirement)
- Two tbsps. of sweet paprika
- One tbsp. of ancho chili powder
- Two tsps. of each
    o Onion powder
    o Garlic powder
- One tsp. of oregano (dried)
- Three-fourth tsp. of each
    o Cumin (ground)
    o Coriander (ground)
    o Nutmeg (grated)
    o Black pepper (ground)

- Two pounds of beef (ground)

- One garlic clove (minced)

- Salt

- Oil (to fry)

- Eight slices of Monterey jack cheese

- Four buns

- Mayonnaise (to serve)

Method:

1. Soak the chili in vinegar for one hour. Drain vinegar and chop the chili.

2. Toast chili powder, paprika, garlic powder, oregano, onion powder, cumin, coriander, nutmeg, and black pepper in a pan.

3. Combine beef with soaked chili, toasted spices, garlic, and salt. Mix well and form four patties.

4. Heat oil in an iron skillet. Sear the patties for five minutes on each side. Add two cheese slices on the patties and cover the skillet. Cook for twenty seconds.

5. Slice the buns. Add mayonnaise on the bun slices. Add the burger patties on each slice of the bun and top with the other half.

Cheese-Chili Burger (La Barra)

Total Prep & Cooking Time: Thirty minutes

Yields: Four servings

Nutrition Facts: Calories: 391.3 | Protein: 34.3g | Carbs: 27.2g| Fat: 12.6g | Fiber: 1.9g

Ingredients

- One pound of ground round
- One cup of plum tomatoes (chopped)
- One-fourth cup of cilantro (minced)
- One tbsp. of chili powder
- Two tsps. of jalapeno pepper (minced)
- Half tsp. of each
    - Salt
    - Oregano
    - Cumin (ground)
- One-fourth tsp. of pepper
- Cooking spray
- Four slices of Monterey jack cheese
- One-third cup of sour cream

- Four hamburger buns

- Four leaves of iceberg lettuce

- Eight tomato slices

Method:

1. Combine the first nine listed ingredients in a large bowl. Make four patties from the mixture.

2. Grill the patties on a grill pan for six minutes on each side. Add one cheese slice on each patty. Grill until the cheese melts.

3. Spread one tbsp. of sour cream on the upper half of the buns. Add the patty on the lower half and top with tomato and lettuce. Add the other half of the bun.

CHAPTER 7:
PASTA RECIPES

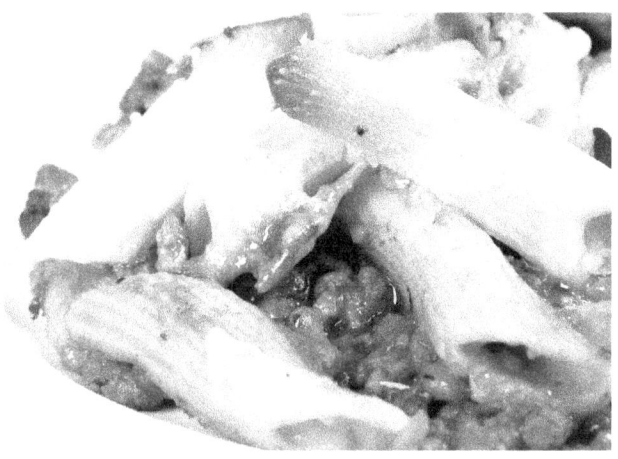

Pasta Skillet (Forno Kapitano)

Total Prep & Cooking Time: Thirty minutes

Yields: Six servings

Nutrition Facts: Calories: 391.3 | Protein: 22.6g | Carbs: 35.6g| Fat: 14.3g | Fiber: 4.2g

Ingredients

- One pound of chuck beef (ground)

- One tsp. of cumin (ground)

- Half tsp. of salt

- Two cups of water

- One can of diced tomatoes (roasted, with chilies)

- Eight ounces of tomato sauce

- Six ounces of pasta (uncooked)

- One and a half cup of Mexican cheese blend

Method:

1. Heat oil in a skillet. Add beef, salt, and cumin. Cook for seven minutes.

2. Add tomatoes, water, tomato sauce, and pasta. Boil the mixture.

3. Cover and simmer for fifteen minutes.

4. Garnish with cheese.

Baked Pasta (Quattro)

Total Prep & Cooking Time: Fifty minutes

Yields: Six servings

Nutrition Facts: Calories: 429.3 | Protein: 23.4g |
Carbs: 37.2g| Fat: 19.5g | Fiber: 3.3g

Ingredients

- One pound of beef (ground)

- One envelope of taco seasoning

- One can of tomato sauce

- One-fourth cup of green pepper
  (chopped)

- One tsp. of garlic powder

- Half tsp. of oregano

- Eight ounces of spiral pasta (cooked)

- One cup of cheddar cheese (shredded)

- Half cup of sour cream

Method:

1. Cook beef in a skillet for five minutes. Add
   tomato sauce, taco seasoning, spices, and
   green pepper. Boil the mixture.

2. Combine a half cup of cheese, sour cream, and pasta in a greased casserole dish. Top with the meat mixture. Sprinkle remaining cheese from the top.

3. Bake for thirty minutes.

Taco Pasta (Dolce Amore)

Total Prep & Cooking Time: Thirty minutes

Yields: Six servings

Nutrition Facts: Calories: 370.3 | Protein: 23.4g | Carbs: 47.5g| Fat: 2.2g | Fiber: 8.6g

Ingredients

- One tbsp. of each
    - o Olive oil
    - o Chili powder
- One pound of chicken (ground)
- One yellow onion (diced)
- One green bell pepper (diced)
- Two garlic cloves (minced)
- One and a half tsp. of cumin (ground)
- Half tsp. of each
    - o Oregano
    - o Salt
- One-fourth tsp. of black pepper (ground)
- One cup of water

- One and a half cup of salsa

- Eight ounces of tomato sauce

- Two cups of whole wheat pasta (uncooked)

- Fifteen ounces of black beans

- Half cup of cheddar cheese (shredded)

Method:

1. Heat oil in a large skillet. Add onion, chicken, and bell peppers. Cook for eight minutes.

2. Add chili powder, garlic, oregano, cumin, salt, and pepper. Cook for one minute. Add water, beans, pasta, and salsa.

3. Simmer for fifteen minutes.

4. Remove from heat. Add cheese and stir.

<u>Chicken Pasta (Rosetta)</u>

Total Prep & Cooking Time: Forty minutes

Yields: Four servings

Nutrition Facts: Calories: 303.2 | Protein: 13.2g | Carbs: 18.5g| Fat: 17.5g | Fiber: 1.1g

Ingredients

- Twelve ounces of spaghetti

- One tbsp. of olive oil

- One pound of chicken breast (cut in pieces of one-inch)

- Salt

- Black pepper (ground)

- One onion (sliced)

- Two bell peppers (sliced)

- One tbsp. of each

  - Cumin (ground)

  - Chili powder

- Two tsps. of oregano

- One can of diced tomatoes

- Half cup of chicken stock

- Three-fourth cup of half and half

- One-third cup of each

  o Cheddar cheese (shredded)

  o Pepper jack cheese (shredded)

- Cilantro (chopped)

Method:

1. Cook the spaghetti by following the package instructions.

2. Heat oil in an iron skillet. Add the chicken. Season with pepper and salt. Cook for six minutes. Add bell peppers and onions. Add the spices and cook for seven minutes.

3. Add stock, half and half, and tomatoes. Cook for three minutes. Add the spaghetti and stir for mixing.

4. Remove from heat and mix the cheeses.

5. Garnish with chopped cilantro.

Mexican One Pot Turkey Pasta (Forno Kapitano)

Total Prep & Cooking Time: Forty minutes

Yields: Six servings

Nutrition Facts: Calories: 370.3 | Protein: 26.3g | Carbs: 28.9g| Fat: 13.6g | Fiber: 4.6g

Ingredients

- Two tsps. of olive oil

- One pound of turkey (ground)

- Half cup of onion (diced)

- Three cloves of garlic (minced)

- Three-fourth tsp. of salt

- One tbsp. of chili powder

- Two tsps. of each

    - Onion powder

    - Garlic powder

    - Cumin (ground)

- Half tsp. of oregano

- Two cups of salsa

- Three cups of water

274

- Two and a half cup of medium shell pasta

- One-third cup of cheddar cheese (shredded)

- Sour cream (to serve)

Method:

1. Preheat your oven at one-hundred and fifty degrees Celsius.

2. Heat oil in an iron skillet. Add the turkey and cook for five minutes; add garlic, onion, and salt. Add garlic powder, chili powder, cumin, onion powder, and oregano. Cook for one minute.

3. Add water, salsa, salt, and pasta. Boil and simmer for ten minutes.

4. Sprinkle cheese from the top.

5. Bake in the oven for two minutes.

6. Use sour cream for garnishing.

Mexican Penne and Avocado (La Posta)

Total Prep & Cooking Time: Forty minutes

Yields: Two servings

Nutrition Facts: Calories: 475.3 | Protein: 14.2g | Carbs: 62.3g| Fat: 14.9g | Fiber: 19.3g

Ingredients

- Hundred grams of penne

- One tsp. of rapeseed oil

- One onion (sliced)

- One orange pepper (cut in chunks)

- Two cloves of garlic (grated)

- Two tsps. of chili powder

- One and a half tsp. of coriander (ground)

- Half tsp. of cumin seeds

- Four-hundred grams of tomatoes (chopped)

- One can of sweet corn

- Two tsps. of vegetable bouillon powder

- One avocado (chopped)

- Half lime (juiced, zested)

Method:

1. Start by cooking penne in salt water for ten minutes. Drain the water.

2. Heat oil in a pan. Add pepper and onion. Add spices and garlic. Cook for twelve minutes. Add tomatoes, water, bouillon, and corn. Simmer for fifteen minutes.

3. Combine avocado along with lime zest and juice in a bowl.

4. Add penne in the sauce and toss.

5. Garnish with avocado.

Mexican Pasta Salad (Dolce Mexico)

Total Prep & Cooking Time: Forty minutes

Yields: Eight servings

Nutrition Facts: Calories: 242.3 | Protein: 11.6g | Carbs: 43.4g| Fat: 3.3g | Fiber: 5.2g

Ingredients

- Four cups of wagon wheel pasta (cooked)

- One can of black beans (rinsed)

- One cup of corn (frozen)

- Half cup of red pepper (chopped)

- Two green onions (sliced)

- One-third cup of ranch dressing

- One tbsp. of taco seasoning mix

- Half tbsp. of lime juice

- One-fourth cup of Mexican cheese blend (shredded)

- Three-fourth cup of cilantro (chopped)

Method:

1. Mix the first five listed ingredients in a large bowl.

2. Combine seasoning mix, dressing, and lime juice; pour it over the salad. Add cilantro and cheese.

3. Toss gently.

CHAPTER 8: JUICE AND DESSERT RECIPES

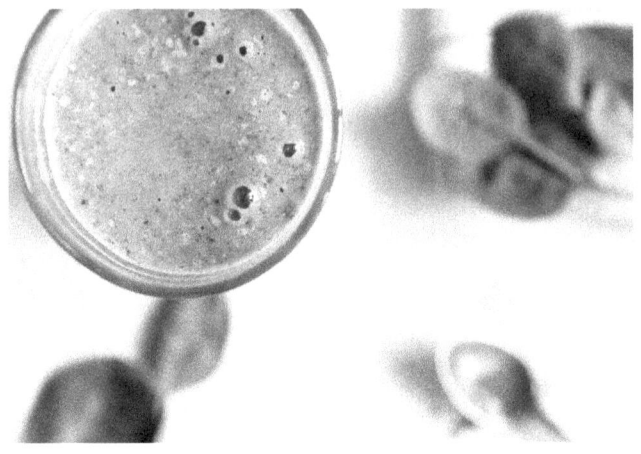

Tres Leches Cake (La Postreria)

Total Prep & Cooking Time: Fifty minutes

Yields: Twenty servings

Nutrition Facts: Calories: 340.2 | Protein: 6.1g | Carbs: 32.6g| Fat: 18.6g | Fiber: 0.6g

Ingredients

- One pack of yellow cake mix

- Three eggs

- Half cup of milk

- One cup of butter (softened)

- One tsp. of vanilla extract

For the topping:

- Fourteen ounces of condensed milk

- One can of evaporated milk

- One and a half cup of whipping cream

For the cream:

- One cup of whipping cream

- Three tbsps. of confectioners' sugar

- One tsp. of vanilla extract

Method:

1. Preheat your oven at one hundred and fifty degrees Celsius.

2. Combine all the cake ingredients in a bowl. Pour in a greased baking dish. Bake for thirty minutes.

3. Combine the listed ingredients for the topping. Poke holes on the cake. Pour the topping. Let sit for twenty minutes.

4. Combine the listed cream ingredients in a bowl. Spread over the cake.

Rice Pudding (Garabatos)

Total Prep & Cooking Time: Forty minutes

Yields: Four servings

Nutrition Facts: Calories: 345.36 | Protein: 7.8g | Carbs: 62.3g| Fat: 6.6g | Fiber: 1.9g

Ingredients

- Two cups of water

- Half cup of long grain rice

- One stick of cinnamon

- One cup of condensed milk

- Three tbsps. of raisins

Method:

1. Combine rice, cinnamon, and water in a pan. Boil the mixture. Simmer for twenty minutes.

2. Add raisins and milk. Simmer for fifteen minutes.

3. Remove the cinnamon.

Sugar Cinnamon Sweet Potato Pastries (Pujol)

Total Prep & Cooking Time: Thirty-five minutes

Yields: Ten servings

Nutrition Facts: Calories: 87.8 | Protein: 1.6g | Carbs: 14.6g| Fat: 5.6g | Fiber: 0.7g

Ingredients

- Half cup of sweet potato (mashed)
- Two ounces of cream cheese (softened)
- One tbsp. of brown sugar
- Half tsp. of orange zest (grated)
- Two tubes of crescent rolls
- Half cup of sugar
- Two tsps. of cinnamon (ground)
- One-fourth cup of butter (melted)

Method:

1. Preheat your oven at one-hundred and fifty degrees Celsius.

2. Mix cream cheese, sweet potato, orange zest, and brown sugar in a bowl.

3. Unroll the rolls and separate into four rectangles. Cut out four triangles from the rectangles. Fill the triangles with sweet potato mixture. Fold to seal.

4. Bake for twelve minutes.

5. Combine cinnamon and sugar in a bowl.

6. Brush the pastries with butter and sprinkle cinnamon mixture.

Watermelon Agua Fresca (Amorino)

Total Prep & Cooking Time: Ten minutes

Yields: Six servings

Nutrition Facts: Calories: 72.3 | Protein: 1.6g | Carbs: 19.6g| Fat: 0.4g | Fiber: 0.9g

Ingredients

- Eights cups of watermelon chunks
- One cup of cold water
- Two tbsps. of each
    - Lime juice
    - Sugar

Method:

1. Combine all the listed ingredients in a high-power food processor. Blend well.
2. Serve cold.

Mexican-Style Strawberry Juice (Quattro)

Total Prep & Cooking Time: Four hours and twenty minutes

Yields: Ten servings

Nutrition Facts: Calories: 99.6 | Protein: 0.6g | Carbs: 22.3g| Fat: 0.1g | Fiber: 1.7g

Ingredients

- Four cups of strawberries (sliced)

- One cup of sugar

- Eight cups of cold water

- One lime (cut in wedges)

- Eight mint sprigs

Method:

1. Combine sugar, one cup of water, and strawberries in a bowl. Refrigerate for four hours.

2. Blend the strawberry mixture with the remaining ingredients except for the lime wedges.

3. Garnish with lime wedges.

Hibiscus Flower Drink (La Postreria)

Total Prep & Cooking Time: Four hours and ten minutes

Yields: Eight servings

Nutrition Facts: Calories: 60.1 | Protein: 0.8g | Carbs: 14.6g| Fat: 0.2g | Fiber: 1.1g

Ingredients

- Two cups of hibiscus Jamaica flowers
- Seven cups of water
- Half cup of sugar
- Ice cubes

Method:

1. Place the hibiscus flowers in a bowl with three cups of water. Boil for two minutes.

2. Keep aside for four hours.

3. Strain the flower liquid in a large pot; add remaining water and sugar. Mix well.

4. Serve with ice cubes.

Mexican Jugo (Rosetta)

Total Prep & Cooking Time: Ten minutes

Yields: Four servings

Nutrition Facts: Calories: 180.3 | Protein: 4.3g | Carbs: 52.6g| Fat: 1.4g | Fiber: 1.3g

Ingredients

- Two cucumbers (sliced)

- Two apples (cubed)

- One bunch of cilantro

- Half green bell pepper (chopped)

- Half lime (with rind)

Method:

1. Process all the listed ingredients in a juicer.

2. Shake for combining.

Green Juice (Thiara)

Total Prep & Cooking Time: Fifteen minutes

Yields: Eight servings

Nutrition Facts: Calories: 96.3 | Protein: 4.3g | Carbs: 18.2g| Fat: 1.1g | Fiber: 7.6g

Ingredients

- Three ounces of spinach

- Two ounces of cucumber (sliced)

- One ounce of each

    o Green bell pepper (sliced)

    o Parsley

    o Celery sliced

- Fifty ounces of orange juice

- Ice cubes (to serve)

Method:

1. Combine all the listed ingredients in a high-power food processor.

2. Chill in the refrigerator for thirty minutes

3. Serve in glasses with ice cubes.

Note: You can use mint leaves for extra flavor.

CONCLUSION

Thank you for making it through to the end of *Copycat Recipes Making*, let's hope it was informative and able to provide you with all of the tools you need to achieve your goals whatever they may be.

Now you can start preparing your favorite dishes mentioned in this book. Keeping aside all the daily meals, the recipes I have included in this book can easily break the monotonous meal routine. You can enjoy all your favorite recipes from the USA and Mexico with no worries at all. If you are looking for an effective way to save money and enjoy your favorite restaurant foods, then copycat recipes are all you need. I hope this book can help you to hone your culinary skills. Now, you can munch on your favorite restaurant snack by preparing the same right in your home kitchen.

If you have reached this page, I believe you are done with checking all the recipes. I have given my best efforts for including the famous recipes from the restaurants, fast food joints, and cities of the USA and Mexico. Hosting a party at your home is no big deal now as you have copycat recipes to your rescue. Not only will you be able to save a lot of money, but you can also keep a check on your overall health. Whether you want to have something from Olive Garden or munch on some snacks from the city of Puebla, this book has got all that you need.

Finally, if you found this book useful in any way, a review on Amazon is always appreciated!

www.ingramcontent.com/pod-product-compliance
Lightning Source LLC
Chambersburg PA
CBHW052308220526
45472CB00001B/29